FEEDING
Tiny Bellies

Lily Payen

FEEDING
Tiny Bellies

Over 100 Baby-Led Weaning, Toddler, and Family Recipes

Foreword by Min Kwon, MS, RDN

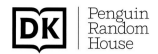

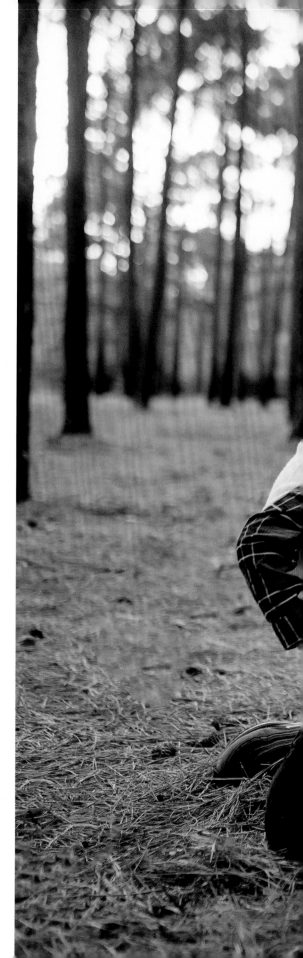

Publisher Mike Sanders
Art & Design Director William Thomas
Editorial Director Ann Barton
Senior Editor Olivia Peluso
Designer Lindsay Dobbs
Food Stylist Petya Baleva
Lifestyle Photographer Candice Fitchett
Recipe Tester Bee Berrie
Copyeditor Christy Wagner
Proofreaders Mira S. Park & Hannah Matuszak
Indexer Louisa Emmons

First American Edition, 2024
Published in the United States by DK Publishing
1745 Broadway, 20th Floor, New York, NY 10019

The authorized representative in the EEA is Dorling Kindersley
Verlag GmbH. Arnulfstr. 124, 80636 Munich, Germany

Copyright © 2024 by Lily Payen
DK, a Division of Penguin Random House LLC
24 25 26 27 28   10 9 8 7 6 5 4 3 2 1
001–340866–Oct/2024

All rights reserved.
Without limiting the rights under the copyright reserved
above, no part of this publication may be reproduced, stored
in or introduced into a retrieval system, or transmitted, in any
form, or by any means (electronic, mechanical, photocopying,
recording, or otherwise), without the prior written permission
of the copyright owner.

A catalog record for this book
is available from the Library of Congress.
ISBN 978-0-7440-9794-8

DK books are available at special discounts when purchased
in bulk for sales promotions, premiums, fund-raising, or
educational use. For details, contact SpecialSales@dk.com

Printed and bound in China

www.dk.com

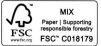

This book was made with Forest
Stewardship Council™ certified
paper – one small step in DK's
commitment to a sustainable future.
Learn more at
www.dk.com/uk/information/sustainability

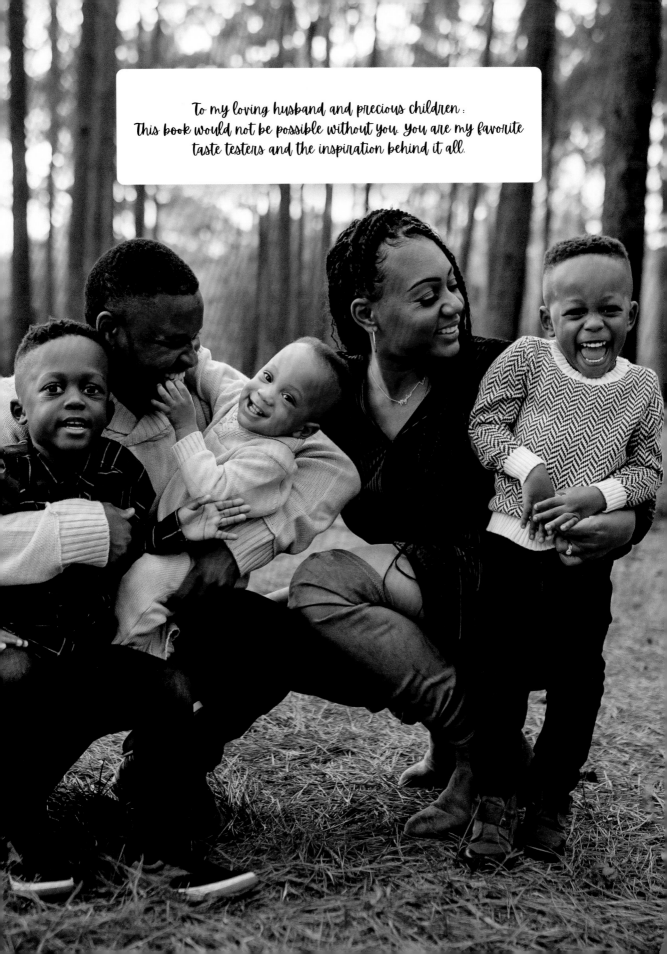

To my loving husband and precious children :
This book would not be possible without you. You are my favorite
taste testers and the inspiration behind it all.

Contents

Snacks & Treats

Sides, Spreads & Dips

Refreshing Drinks

Foreword

Whether you're a first-time mom nervously embarking on the exciting milestone of starting your child on solid foods or a seasoned parent, feeding babies can present its share of challenges. From figuring out how to introduce solid foods in a safe and nutritious manner to guiding your little one to embrace a variety of flavors and textures, mealtime with babies can be both joyful and overwhelming.

But don't worry! This true gem of a book by Lily, a dedicated mom of three, is here to empower and guide you through this journey. Having experienced firsthand the struggles that come with introducing solids to little ones, Lily has committed herself to developing nutritious and scrumptious recipes that not only cater to your baby's growth and development needs but also make mealtimes a delightful experience for the entire family.

As a pediatric registered dietitian, I am thrilled that each of Lily's recipes focuses on including the vital nutrients that babies need to grow and thrive. From iron-rich ingredients to healthy fats essential for brain development, every bite is thoughtfully designed to make it count.

And as a busy mom myself, I value how simple and straightforward these recipes are. They guarantee that you can nourish your little one without adding extra stress to your already bustling life.

As you flip through these pages packed with wholesome and tasty recipes, you'll find that you're not just exploring a book on baby-led weaning. You are setting out on a delightful and heartwarming adventure that will ignite your little one's taste buds and create everlasting memories at the family table.

And as much as we all want our babies to devour everything, the reality is that they will need a generous dose of patience, love, and gentle encouragement to master this new skill that takes time to learn. So if your baby doesn't immediately take to the meals you prepare, don't be disheartened. Remember, you are introducing them to a world of flavors and textures, which is essential for laying the foundation for becoming adventurous eaters.

So let's press on! We are all in this together.

Min Kwon, MS, RDN

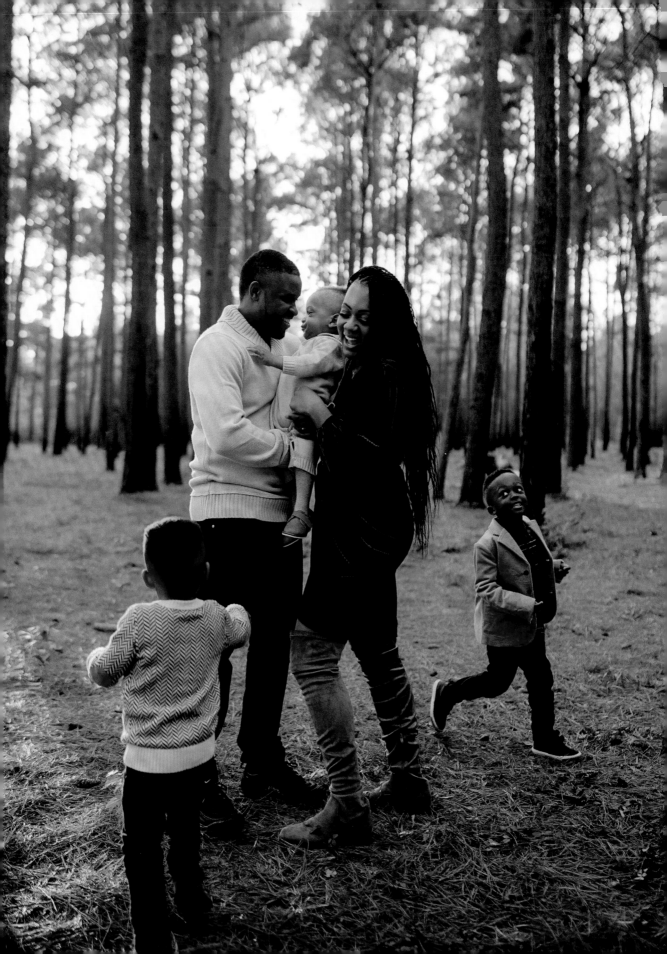

Introduction

Hi and welcome! I'm Lily, the mama behind Feeding Tiny Bellies, and I'm here to help you take some of the stress out of mealtimes for your little ones.

I'm a busy mom of three and still vividly remember how overwhelmed I felt when it came time to offer my first son, Myles, solids. I was lost on where to start, what to feed him, and how to balance making meals for the entire family. I started out by offering him purees, which he hated and spat out every single time. I spent so much time trying to get creative, blending different fruit and vegetable combinations and freezing them in batches, only for him to hate them all. He just wasn't into purees. I did notice that he was always so attentive whenever my husband and I were having a meal at the table. One day, I decided to give him a little taste of what we were eating. I'd never seen him put something into his mouth so eagerly. I handed him another piece, and he gobbled it up. That was the moment I realized he wanted to eat what we eat!

I no longer had to spend so much time making separate meals for him. He could explore all the flavors and textures of the meals we prepared for ourselves. I shifted my focus to creating family-centered meals and modifying them for him to enjoy as well. This took off so much pressure—we were finally able to enjoy meals together.

Two years later, I gave birth to my second son, Levi. I immediately knew that I wanted to jump into baby-led weaning when he turned six months old, but he was born at a crazy time, during a pandemic when grocery store runs weren't as easy to do. I still wanted to create nutritious meals for him, but I was limited to the basic staples I had in my fridge and pantry. I aimed to create simple recipes with simple ingredients that were still filling and balanced—because meals don't have to be complicated to be nutritious!

Feeding kids can be hard! Sometimes, life gets busy, and it feels impossible to manage everything around us. Getting balanced meals on the table is another thing to add to the list of seemingly never-ending tasks. If you're a busy parent, you likely won't have time to make separate, elaborate meals for your baby. This book contains simple, tasty, and nutritious recipes that are designed for babies and toddlers but with the whole family in mind. Each recipe includes tips for modifying and safely serving portions for babies. With this book, you can make quick and nutritious meals for the whole family, without having to labor for hours in the kitchen!

I'll guide you through the most commonly asked questions for navigating the weaning journey. I'll provide sane advice for picky eaters and the common stages they go through as their appetites change and they grow from babies into toddlerhood. And I'll share time-saving cooking tips and tricks to help you manage your time more effectively. Let this book be your one-stop shop for creating delicious recipes that the whole family will love as well as your trusted guide for navigating the challenges and successes that come with *feeding tiny bellies*!

Lily Payen

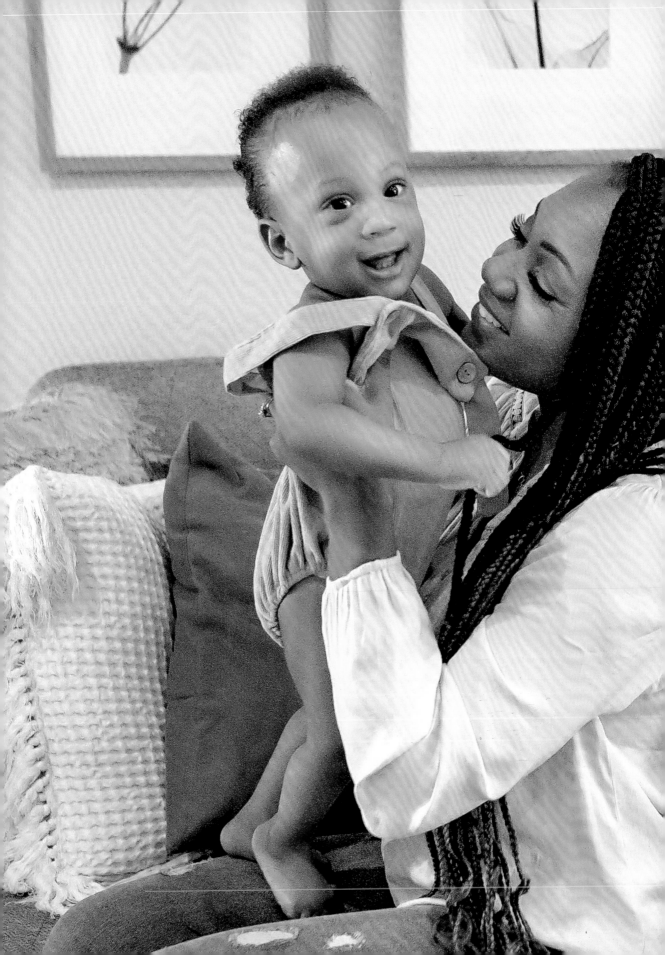

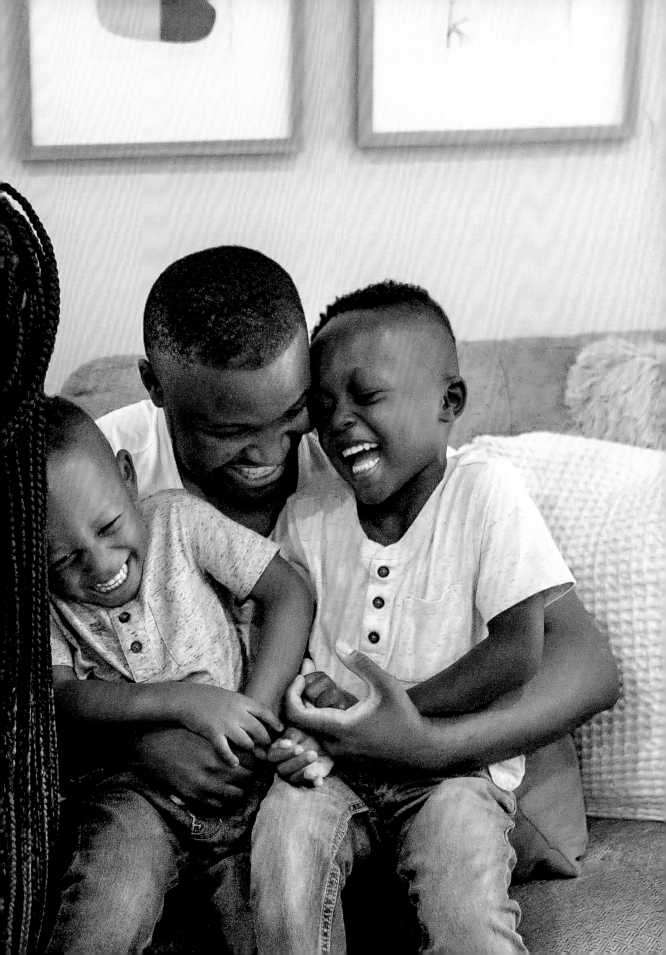

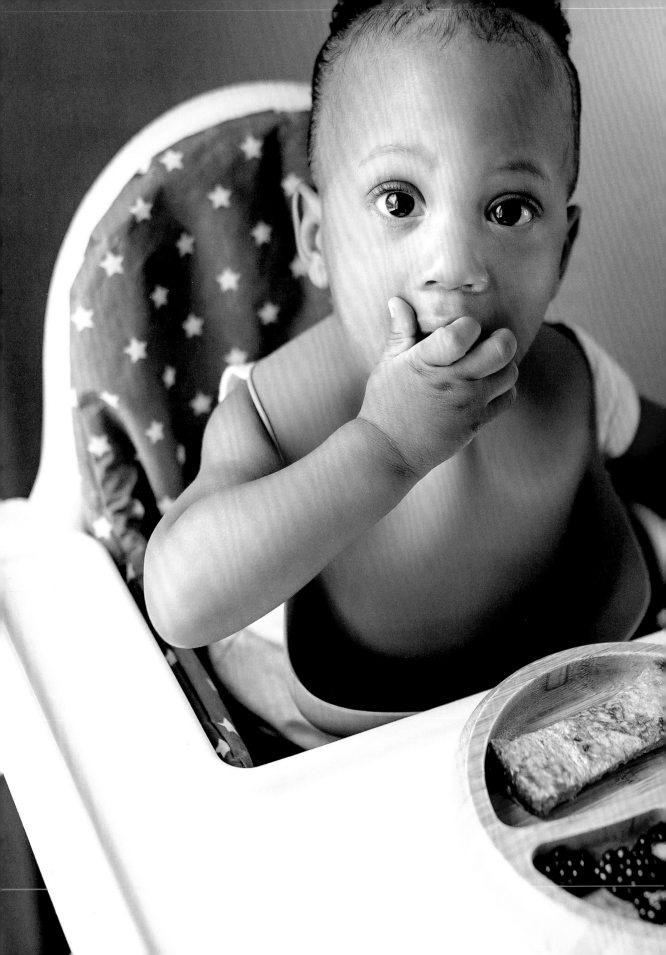

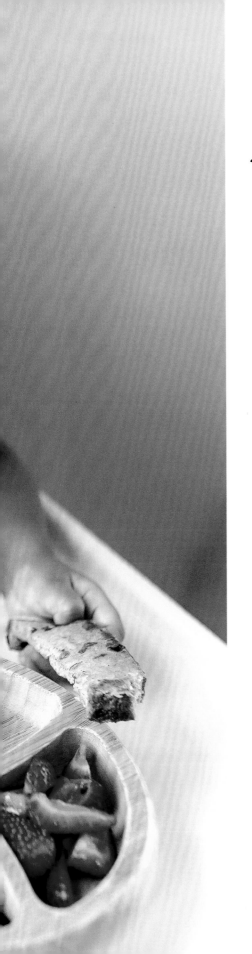

A Guide to Baby-Led Weaning

Baby-led weaning (BLW) has gained a lot of popularity in the past few years, but what exactly does it entail? Where do you start? What are the benefits? In this chapter, I'll unpack all the basics about this method of introducing solid foods, including signs of readiness, what you'll need, how to serve meals, foods to avoid, and how BLW can be worked into your family's life. Whether you're far along into your BLW journey or you're just hearing about it for the first time, this chapter will guide you through it all.

What Is Baby-Led Weaning?

Baby-led weaning (BLW) is a feeding approach for introducing solids to babies. The term was coined in 2008 by Gill Rapley, PhD, the founding philosopher of the BLW method, and has been steadily gaining popularity since. With this approach, a baby jumps straight into self-feeding when they start eating solid foods rather than being spoon-fed purees. These foods can be finger foods and foods with a variety of textures. Baby is encouraged to explore foods independently and take full control when eating. It can be a little overwhelming to comprehend at first, so let's break down the basics.

What Are the Benefits and Challenges of Baby-Led Weaning?

Before you start BLW, it's important to consider the benefits and challenges so you're prepared for what may come your way.

Benefits

- **BLW saves time:** With BLW, there's no need to create separate meals because baby can eat the same foods the rest of the family eats (with slight modifications). This promotes early integration into family meals.

- **BLW helps babies learn to self-regulate:** Baby can control how much food to eat and is able to stop when full.

- **BLW can reduce picky eating:** With BLW, baby experiences tasting a large variety of food textures and consistencies, which may help them develop an appreciation for different foods and hopefully reduce picky eating down the line.

- **BLW helps babies learn coordination:** BLW is excellent for helping baby practice coordination. Baby consistently practices hand-eye coordination and chewing skills during mealtimes.

- **BLW promotes independence:** Baby is able to select what and how much they want to eat and develop a sense of independence at an early age.

Challenges

- **BLW can be messy:** Giving babies the liberty to self-feed can be messier than spoon-feeding! Fortunately, there are things that can help with overcoming the mess.

- **BLW can cause food waste:** Oftentimes, some food goes to waste, especially during the food-dropping stage (see page 38). Keeping portions small to start can definitely help reduce waste.

- **BLW can cause gagging:** Gagging may occur, especially in the initial stages. This may cause parents to worry, but gagging is a normal mechanism babies use as a defense against choking, and thankfully, it gets better with time.

What Are the Signs of Readiness to Begin Baby-Led Weaning?

Before you begin BLW with your little one, look out for these signs of readiness:

- Baby is at least six months of age.

- Baby can sit up unassisted with little to no support.

- Baby has demonstrated good head control.

- Baby's tongue-thrust reflex (the reflex that causes a baby to push objects out of their mouth to prevent choking) begins to disappear.

- Baby has developed the coordination to be able to pick up objects and bring them to their mouth.

- Baby shows interest in solid foods.

How to Serve Foods

BLW encourages baby to eat what you eat, so there's no need to make separate "baby food." But it is important to note that foods must be cut appropriately before they're considered safe to offer to baby.

Beginners have something called the palmar grasp. They will use their entire hand to pick up objects, and they are able to curl their fingers around an object in the palm of their hand. Foods cut into finger-length strips are easy for babies to pick up using their whole hand. Finger-length strips also help your baby learn how to take appropriate bites and chew. Most babies will only be able to access the part of the food that is sticking out of their closed fist, so don't expect your little one to finish the whole strip of food at this stage.

As they grow, babies develop something called the pincer grasp: They will be able to pick up small objects with their index fingers and thumbs. This usually happens between nine and twelve months of age. After your baby develops their pincer grasp, you may begin to offer foods cut into smaller pieces. For round objects, such as blueberries, smash or quarter them to remove the roundness.

Baby-Led Weaning Essentials

When it comes to BLW, you don't need much, but here are some basic essentials to get you started. These items aren't all must-haves, but some of them are good to have to make the process a little easier.

- **High chair:** A high chair is a must-have and important to ensure that baby sits in a stable, comfortable, and safe position. Opt for a high chair with a footrest (or one that has the capability to add an adjustable footrest) so your baby's feet are firmly planted when they are seated. Baby should be sitting upright or leaning forward slightly, not reclined, with a ninety-degree bend at the hips, knees, and ankles. This helps stabilize their core and supports safe swallows.

- **Bibs:** Bibs keep baby as clean as possible during mealtimes. Silicone bibs with front pockets are great for catching food items that may fall as your baby brings them to their mouth. Depending on the food offered, you also can strip your baby down to their diaper for easy cleanup!

- **Strong suction plates:** These plates are difficult for baby to remove from their high chair tray, meaning more food stays on the plate. Alternatively, you may choose to skip plates and place food directly on the high chair tray.

- **Utensils:** Babies can use utensils after they shift from primarily using their hands to eat. Short-handled spoons are great for when baby is eating pureed, textured foods such as yogurt and applesauce. These foods can be preloaded onto a spoon for your little one to self-feed. Many utensils also double as teethers to help soothe gums.

- **Cups:** Cups help baby practice hand-eye coordination when consuming liquids.

What Foods Should You Start With?

When introducing solids, certain foods are better to start with than others. You want foods than can be portioned into finger foods, either cut into finger-length strips and easily smashable or served whole if they are larger than the size of baby's mouth.

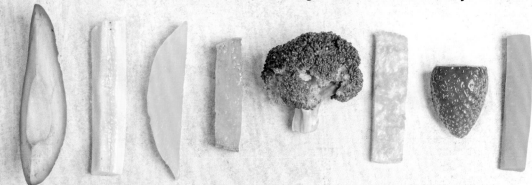

- Avocado slice
- Banana slice
- Mango slice

- Roasted sweet potato slice
- Steamed broccoli floret
- Cooked egg strip

- Large ripe strawberry
- Steamed carrot slice

If you find that your baby is struggling to pick up some of these foods, you can try coating them in some ground seeds, almond flour, or unsweetened shredded coconut for some texture. You also can leave on a bit of the food's skin to help with added grip. Depending on the food, be sure to take away the food or peel it when they get to the skin, so they don't eat it. You can use a crinkle cutter when cutting slippery foods to provide texture and grip.

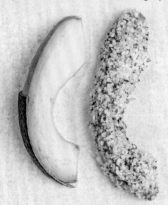
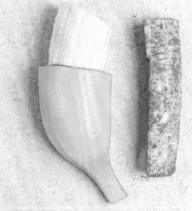
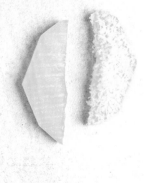

- **Avocados:** Leave a little bit of the skin on or coat with hemp hearts to provide a little grip.

- **Bananas:** Lightly score the peel from a piece of a banana to remove that part of the peel and expose part of the banana. Leaving some of the peel on the bottom provides a handle for babies to grip. Alternatively, you may coat a piece of banana in ground flaxseeds to provide some grip.

- **Mangoes:** Use a crinkle cutter to slice a mango to add some ridged edges for texture. You may also coat a mango slice in unsweetened shredded coconut for some added grip.

After your baby develops the pincer grasp, you can begin to offer small, bite-size pieces of food. This doesn't mean you should completely abandon serving foods in strips, but you should try to give your baby plenty of practice developing and mastering their pincer grasp. You can modify those same first foods when your baby has developed the pincer grasp.

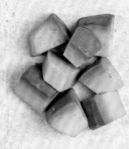

- Diced avocado

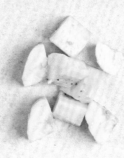

- Diced banana

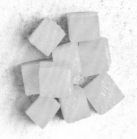

- Diced mango

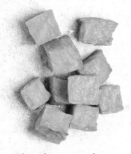

- Diced roasted sweet potatoes

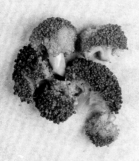

- Chopped steamed broccoli florets

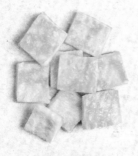

- Diced cooked egg strip

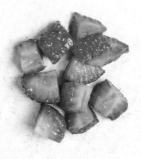

- Diced strawberry

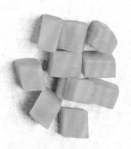

- Diced steamed carrot

Introducing Allergens

In 2000, the American Academy of Pediatrics (AAP) recommended delaying the introduction of high-allergenic foods to babies for the first one to three years of life. In 2008, the AAP updated its guidelines, stating that the introduction of allergens should not be delayed. The US Department of Agriculture's (USDA's) 2020–2025 Dietary Guidelines for Americans (DGA) now show that there is no benefit to delaying the introduction of allergenic foods.[1] In fact, that approach seems to be counterproductive. Most experts believe that exposure to allergenic foods early and often can reduce the potential for food allergies.

When introducing top allergens, it's a good idea to offer them one at a time along with nonallergenic foods. For example, do not offer eggs and peanuts in the same meal for first exposure because they are both top allergens. Introducing potential allergens independently helps you better watch for reactions and pinpoint exact triggers.

Here are the top nine allergenic foods that make up about 90 percent of all allergens:

- Dairy
- Eggs
- Peanuts
- Tree nuts
- Fish
- Shellfish
- Soy
- Wheat
- Sesame

When introducing common allergens, keep track of any symptoms your baby displays that seem unusual. Some common symptoms of allergic reactions include the following:

- Widespread hives
- Itchiness
- Swelling of the lips or tongue
- Redness of the skin
- Dry cough
- Nausea or vomiting
- Diarrhea
- Shortness of breath or wheezing
- Difficulty swallowing
- Change in skin color

If you notice that your baby is displaying any of these symptoms, stop serving the food item and immediately reach out to your child's pediatrician or health-care provider or seek medical help right away. If you think your child is having a severe allergic reaction with compromised breathing or severe swelling, it's an emergency. Call 911 or go to the nearest emergency room immediately.

Portion Sizes

What portion sizes should you offer your baby? It varies! There is no right answer here. A portion that is overwhelming for one baby may be underwhelming for another. Every baby is different.

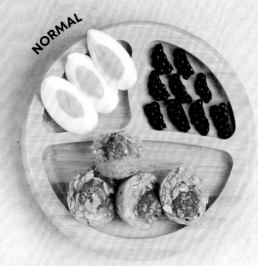

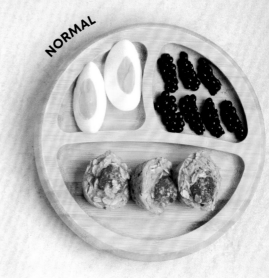

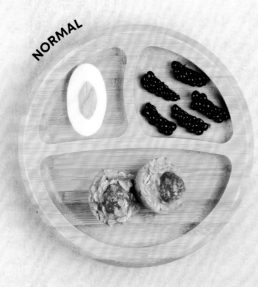

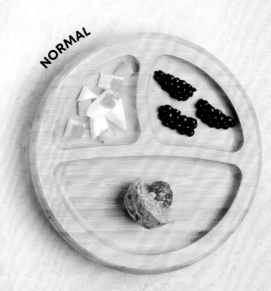

Start with small portions, and offer more if your baby seems interested. This eliminates potential food waste and helps baby not feel too overwhelmed initially. Once you get a sense of the portion size your baby does best with, you can follow their lead.

As long as your baby is following their growth curve, they are consuming the right amount for what their body needs.

Meal Frequency

We often hear that the goal is to get to three meals and two snacks a day by age one, but how exactly do we get there? As with portion sizes, there is no right answer here, either. There is no one-size-fits-all guide when it comes to introducing meals. Babies are so different and progress at varied paces. Some are ready to move to two meals a day within weeks of beginning solids, while others need months. Follow your baby's lead when it comes to introducing meals. Start slow with just one meal a day to give your baby's digestive system time to adjust from a milk-only diet of breast milk or formula, and work your way up from there.

What Course Should You Start With?

Breakfast, lunch, or dinner—it's your choice! The type of food doesn't matter as much as the variety of foods offered. When it comes to offering a meal, pick a time when your baby is happy and relaxed. Opt for a time when the meal won't be rushed.

What About Milk?

Continue offering the same amount of milk until the age of one. Breast milk or formula should remain the main source of nutrition for the first twelve months of life. The AAP and World Health Organization (WHO) recommend continuing breastfeeding for up to two years of age, but generally, milk intake decreases after age one.

What If Baby Prefers Milk Over Solids?

That's normal! Transitioning to solid foods is a brand-new experience for babies. It may take them some time to adjust to solids being a part of their diet.

What If Baby Prefers Solids Over Milk?

That's also normal! Continue to offer the same amount of milk (breast milk or formula) so baby can adjust to both. Solid foods are needed at six months to help meet nutrient needs (see page 32 for more), but they should complement the primarily milk-based diet for the first twelve months. Speak to your child's pediatrician if you are concerned that their milk intake is too low.

Flavoring Food for Babies

The Centers for Disease Control and Prevention (CDC) and England's National Health Service (NHS) recommend that added salt should be avoided for babies under age one,[2] but this doesn't mean that their food should lack flavor! Salt-free seasonings and spices are excellent ways of flavoring foods and expanding your little one's palate.

Introduce different seasonings into your baby's foods to see what they like. Don't assume that your little one doesn't like a certain spice or seasoning if they spit it out the first time. Tasting a new flavor is an unfamiliar experience for your child, so you may need to offer an item multiple times for them to get accustomed to it and learn to appreciate its taste. There also may be instances when your baby doesn't like a certain spice or flavor, and that's okay! We all have our favorites, so it's perfectly acceptable if your little one develops some taste preferences as well.

Added Sugars

The CDC and NHS also recommend avoiding added sugars for babies and using natural sweeteners instead.[2] Fruits are amazing natural sweeteners. Overripe bananas make great sweeteners and binders in recipes, and ripe berries add sweetness and a slight tartness. Dates, raisins, and maple syrup are also good refined-sugar-free replacements in baked goods. They are higher in sugar content compared to bananas and berries, but they are naturally concentrated sugars.

You will notice throughout the recipes in this book that maple syrup is used as a sweetener in some baked goods. If you prefer to use a fruit-based sweetener, you can replace the maple syrup in those recipes with mashed banana or unsweetened applesauce in a 1:1 ratio.

Spices & Seasonings

Many of the recipes in this book use spices and seasonings to add flavor for our little ones to enjoy. Here are some great staples to have on hand to incorporate into any recipe:

- Black pepper
- Chili powder
- Cinnamon (ground)
- Cumin (ground)
- Garlic powder
- Ginger (ground)
- Italian seasoning
- Nutmeg (ground)
- Onion powder
- Oregano (dried)
- Parsley (dried)
- Pumpkin pie spice
- Sweet paprika
- Vanilla extract

Remember, you can always add salt to foods for the rest of the family after removing baby's portion.

Important Nutrients for Babies & Toddlers

When your little one reaches six months old, there are some crucial nutrients that they need to get from foods. Offering a balanced diet helps meet these needs, but certain nutrients are worth paying special attention to because they are very important for baby's development.

Iron

Children need iron for their brains and bodies to develop properly. Iron allows blood cells to carry oxygen to all parts of the body, which is crucial for development. A newborn baby has enough iron to support growth for the first few months of life. From seven through twelve months of age, recommended iron intake increases from 0.3 milligrams (mg) per day to 11 mg per day. This is a pretty significant jump, so it's important to offer iron-rich foods to help your baby maximize iron absorption. It can be overwhelming to try to "meet" that goal, but keep in mind this is just a recommendation and appetites vary from day to day. Try not to focus on counting the milligrams, and instead try to offer iron sources with all meals.

Here are some ways to increase iron intake:

- Offer an iron source at every meal. There are two different types of iron: heme iron and nonheme iron. Heme iron is found in animal sources, like meat, poultry, and fish. Nonheme iron is found in plant foods, like whole grains, beans, and leafy greens. Nonheme iron is less absorbable than heme iron, but there are ways to boost absorption of both forms.

- Pair the source of iron with a source of vitamin C to assist in iron absorption. This technique is especially beneficial for nonheme iron sources, which are not naturally well absorbed. Choosing a fruit or veggie to serve at each meal is an excellent way to incorporate vitamin C.

- Cook foods in a cast-iron pan. This is a safe way to add iron to cooked dishes.

Zinc

Zinc is an important mineral for growth, immune function, wound healing, and development of proper taste and smell. Our bodies cannot store zinc effectively, so it's important to consistently offer zinc-rich foods to little ones. Thankfully, zinc and iron share common food sources, so your child is likely meeting their zinc needs if they are consistently offered iron-rich foods.

Omega-3 Fatty Acids

Docosahexaenoic acid (DHA) and eicosapentaenoic acid (EPA) are types of omega-3 fatty acids that are needed to help support brain growth and function. Our bodies cannot produce them, so it is important to ensure that your child consumes foods rich in fatty acids to meet these needs. Oily fish, like salmon, and omega-3-rich eggs are great options for fatty acids.

Building a Balanced Plate

Black Beans, Strawberry, and Avocado
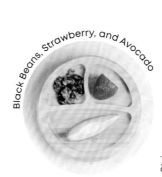

Egg Strip, Raspberries, and Buttered Toast Strip
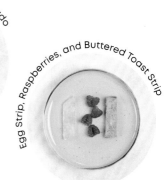

Rice Ball, Broccoli, and Salmon
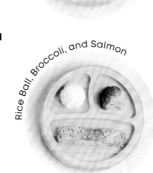

Chicken, Quinoa, and Sweet Potato Strip
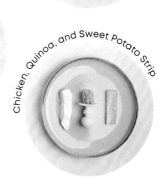

When creating a balanced meal for a baby or toddler, follow this basic formula to ensure you include each of the following in their meals:

1. A source of iron
2. A source of vitamin C (fruit or vegetable)
3. A high-calorie energy source

Some foods may fit into more than one category, which is great!

Iron Sources

Sources of heme iron include beef meatballs, chicken breasts, chicken drumsticks, ground turkey, lamb chops, pork roast, salmon, sardines, shrimp, and tuna.

Sources of nonheme iron include chickpeas (garbanzo beans), edamame, eggs, hemp hearts, kidney beans, lentils, oatmeal, quinoa, spinach, and tofu.

Vitamin C Sources

Sources of vitamin C include bell peppers, broccoli, cauliflower, grapefruit, kiwi, limes, mangoes, oranges, strawberries, and tomatoes.

High-Calorie Energy Sources

High-calorie energy sources include avocados, coconut milk, flaxseeds, full-fat cheeses, nut butters, olive oil, pasta, salmon, seed butters, and whole-grain bread.

The following table offers some good examples of balanced plates that include iron, vitamin C, and high-calorie energy sources.

Balanced Plate Examples

Iron Source	Vitamin C Source	High Calorie/ Energy Dense
Beef Meatballs	Tomato Sauce	Pasta
Black Beans	Strawbery	Avocado Slice
Oatmeal	Banana Slices	Peanut Butter (mixed into oatmeal)
Egg Strip	Raspberries	Buttered Toast Strip
Chicken Strip	Sweet Potato Strip	Quinoa
Salmon	Broccoli	Rice Ball

Remember, it is our job as parents to offer diverse, nutrient-rich foods, but it's our little one's job to decide what and how much to eat. It's okay if your child only ends up eating one of the foods you offer. Balance is achieved over time.

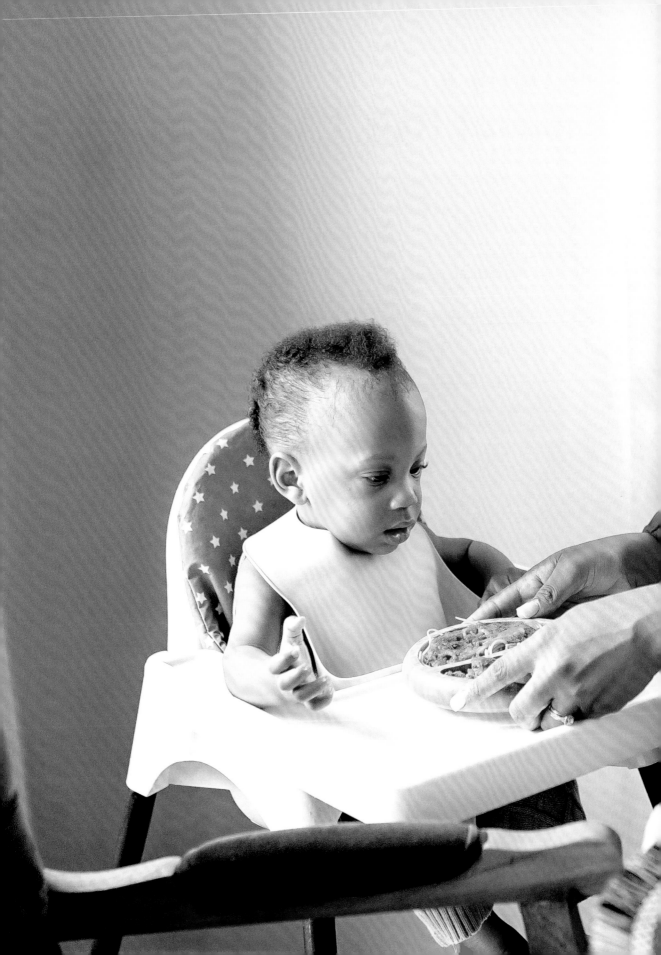

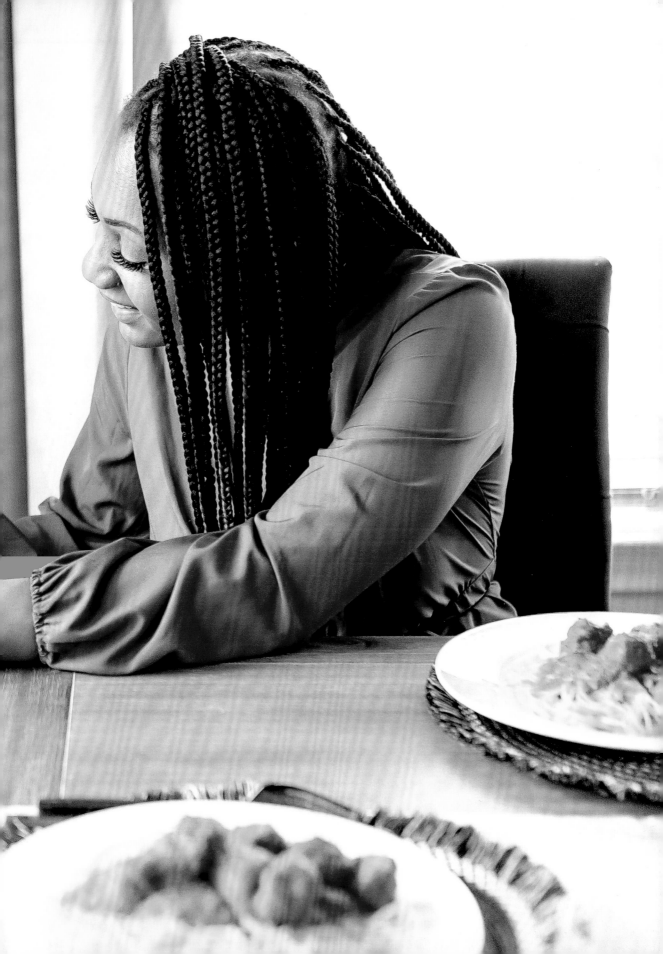

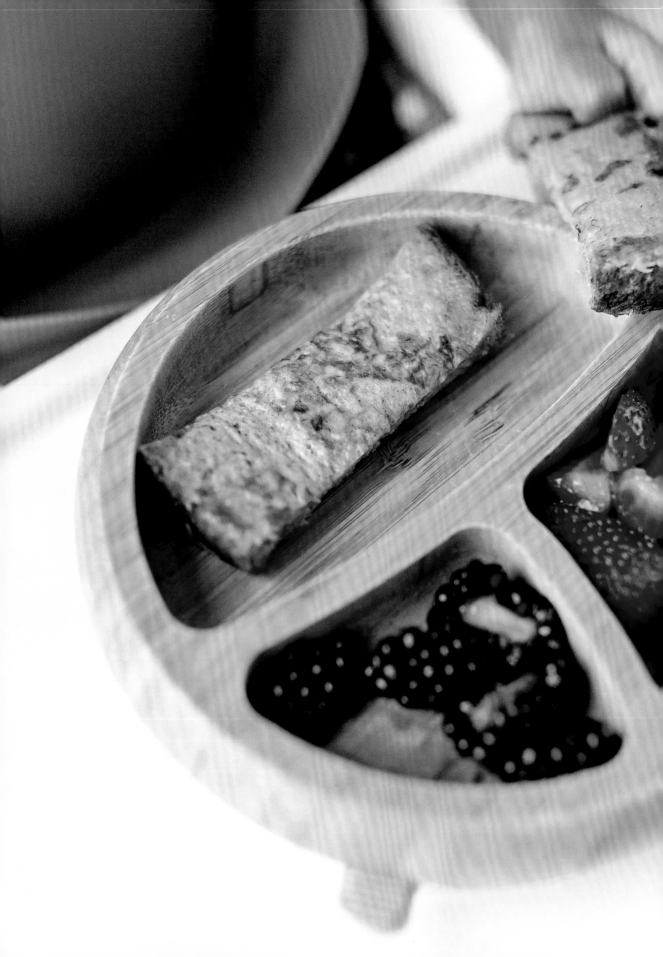

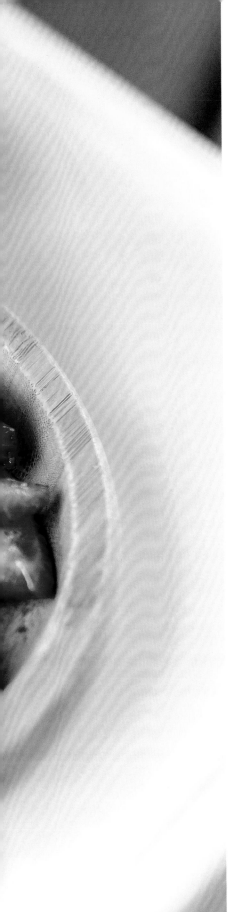

Common Baby-Led Weaning Myths

Introducing solids to your baby is an exciting time, but that excitement can easily turn into anxiety when you're bombarded with information and opinions and it's hard to tell what's true or false. There is so much conflicting advice and so many outdated tips regarding introducing solids, so in this chapter, we'll take a look at some common myths and discover what's actually true.

15 Baby-Led Weaning Myths

Many parents and caregivers can easily feel overwhelmed when it comes to starting solids, with so much information floating around about the "right" and "wrong" ways to go about it. Let's debunk some common feeding myths with evidence-based information so you can feel more confident jumping into this feeding journey with your little one!

Myth 1: Babies Need Teeth to Eat Finger Foods

Babies do not need teeth to eat finger foods. Babies' gums are so strong (if your baby has ever accidentally bitten down on your finger, you know just how strong those little gums can be!) and can tackle several textures. As adults, we chew and break down foods with our back molars, not our front teeth. The first teeth that babies get are their front top and bottom teeth, and those teeth are not for chewing anyway. Babies are quite capable of mashing and grinding up all types of foods with their gums. Keep in mind that foods should be soft, easily mashable, and appropriately sized and served according to your baby's age. The general rule is that if you can easily squish a food between your index finger and thumb, it is generally safe to offer to your baby. You'll be surprised at what those little gums can do!

Myth 2: Baby Food Needs to Be Bland

Many people think that a lack of salt results in a lack of flavor, but that is definitely not the case. Baby food does not need to be bland! There are so many ways to season and flavor foods for babies without adding salt. Babies are actually born with more taste buds than adults, and they can develop taste preferences in the womb, so it's important to introduce a variety of flavors early on. New studies have shown that this can help create a more complex palate in children.

So how can you flavor food for your baby? Natural spices are a great way to enhance and add flavor to different dishes. Cinnamon, nutmeg, and ginger can enhance the natural sweetness of baked goods. Garlic powder, onion powder, black pepper, and paprika can enhance savory recipes. All of these spices and more (see page 23) are packed with flavor that can make a dish tasty for your little one without added sugar or salt.

Myth 3: Babies Are More Likely to Choke with Baby-Led Weaning

Choking is a very common concern parents have when it comes to introducing solids. It is a very serious worry, but don't let that fear hold you back from offering a variety of foods to your baby. Studies have shown that baby-led weaning (BLW) is not associated with an increased risk of choking and that there is no increased risk in choking episodes between those fed traditional purees versus those fed BLW style.[3] Certain foods need to be prepared in specific ways before they should be offered to your little ones to reduce the risk of choking. Some common choking hazards include, but aren't limited to, whole blueberries, popcorn, raw carrots, hot dogs, and globs of peanut butter. The Centers for Disease Control and Prevention (CDC) website offers an extensive list of choking hazards for babies and toddlers.[4]

Choking Versus Gagging

It is very common to mistake gagging for choking. It's essential that you know the difference between the two so you know when to intervene. It can be nerve-wracking to watch your baby gag, but it is a normal part of learning how to eat. The gag reflex is a built-in response that prevents large objects from entering the airway, and it is farther up in the mouth in babies than in adults. As babies get older, it moves farther back, but gagging is very common in the first few weeks of starting solid foods. During a gag, your baby is actively working to spit out a piece of food. During a choke, a baby's airway is partly or completely blocked, meaning that they are not able to breathe properly.

If your child is gagging, do not intervene. Remain calm and let your child work out the food. If you panic and try to insert your fingers into baby's mouth, that can actually lead to choking.

Signs of gagging:

- The child's mouth is open and their tongue is thrust forward.

- The child is coughing and/or sputtering.

- The child's face may appear red.

Signs of choking:

- The child may be wheezing or unable to produce sounds.

- The child is silent or has a weak cough.

- The child's face appears blue or gray.

If your child is choking, intervention is needed *immediately.*

I highly recommend taking an infant cardiopulmonary resuscitation (CPR) course so that you are prepared in case of a choking emergency. Offering appropriately cut foods and waiting for signs of readiness reduces the risk of choking, but it is always best to be prepared. Taking a CPR course will also help reduce your anxiety at mealtimes.

If you feel like your baby is gagging more than normal on a particular food, skip it and try it again after your baby's chewing and self-feeding skills improve. At the end of the day, trust your instincts: If a certain food makes you feel nervous, offer it when both you and your baby feel ready.

Tips to Avoid Choking

Here are some tips to help prevent choking:

- Never leave your child unattended while they're eating.

- Ensure that your child is sitting in an appropriate upright position and that their back is straight.

- Model safe eating habits and chewing food thoroughly before swallowing.

- Avoid distractions while your child is eating. Be sure your child is not running or playing while eating because sudden movements can be dangerous.

- Offer liquids as needed.

- Always consider the shape, size, consistency, and texture of a food before offering it to your little one.

Myth 4: Babies Can Eat Everything You Can Eat

Babies can eat and handle textures of many of the same foods you eat yourself, but there are some foods that are not safe and should be avoided and other foods that should be offered in moderation. The following list outlines foods to avoid or offer only in moderation:

- **Honey:** Honey should not be given to babies under the age of one due to the risk of infant botulism. Honey is often added to many prepackaged items, so be sure to read food labels carefully before offering something to your baby.

- **Meats, eggs, and seafood:** Meats, eggs, and seafood should be fully cooked for children under the age of five. Beef, pork, and lamb should be cooked to a minimum of 145°F (65°C), and poultry should be cooked to a minimum of 165°F (75°C) per the American Academy of Pediatrics (AAP).[5]

- **Unpasteurized dairy:** Unpasteurized milk or cheese is not safe for babies. Unpasteurized products can be contaminated with bacteria and other disease-causing organisms and should be avoided.

- **Choking hazards:** Foods like popcorn, hard candies, and chunks of raw, hard vegetables are choking hazards and should be avoided. Please see the CDC's website for an extensive list of choking hazards.[4]

- **Salt:** Babies and toddlers only need a very small amount of salt in their diets, and babies get most of this from breast milk or formula. Avoid offering foods that are high in salt. When cooking a meal for the entire family, remove your baby's portion first, before adding salt to the remaining meal.

- **Sugar:** The CDC and the National Health Service (NHS) recommend avoiding added sugars for children under the age of two.[2] Certain things are fine to offer in moderation, but there are several ways to sweeten food with natural sugars from fruits instead of sugar. Many babies and toddlers are content with foods that are naturally sweetened. It is likely that your little one will consume foods containing added sugar before age two, and that is perfectly fine. It's good to be mindful, but an occasional taste of foods with added sugar won't hurt.

Myth 5: Baby-Led Weaning Is the Best Way to Wean Your Baby

There is no "best" way to wean your baby. There is no "best" way for your baby to learn about foods and textures. There is no "best" way for your little one to be introduced to and progress with solid food. Every baby is different and has unique needs. Some families prefer to start their babies with traditional purees, while others jump straight into serving finger foods. Regardless of the feeding approach that you choose for your baby, the end goal is the same: for your baby to develop the skills needed to eat a variety of foods, to have a diversified and balanced diet, and to enjoy eating!

Myth 6: Food Before One Is Just for Fun

This is a common phrase you may hear as you begin to introduce foods to your little one. Food before age one can be fun, but it isn't *just* for fun. It is true that breast milk or formula is and should remain a baby's main source of nutrition until age one, but it is also true that solid food holds importance starting at six months of age. Solid foods are needed to meet your little one's necessary nutrient needs. This is especially important for iron-rich foods because breast milk and formula do not contain enough iron to meet your baby's iron needs after six months of age. Introducing solid foods is also important for developmental, motor, and coordination skills. The spirit of the phrase is lighthearted (don't stress about the quantity of food your baby consumes!), but exposure to solid foods is necessary and important.

Myth 7: You Should Stop Offering Foods Your Baby Doesn't Like

When you are first beginning solids with your little one, you may notice that all they do is squish and play with the food that you've prepared. They may take small bites and make faces of disgust, but this is normal. Starting solids can be a huge adjustment for a baby who has had nothing but milk for months. Experiencing different textures and tastes is a big change, and it's a normal part of the exploration process. If your baby doesn't seem interested in a certain type of food, keep offering it. It sometimes can take several times of reoffering a food for a baby to try it. Does this mean that if you reintroduce a food several times, your little one is bound to love it one day? No. Just as we adults have likes and dislikes, babies and toddlers have preferences, too. But exposure to different foods and textures is just as important as actually consuming them.

Myth 8: Babies Should Not Have Dairy Before Age One

Breast milk, formula, or water (water specifically from six months old) should be the only liquids provided for the first year of life, yet this doesn't mean that babies shouldn't have dairy. Dairy in small amounts in baked goods or recipes is absolutely allowed. Dairy in foods like cheese and yogurt is also perfectly fine to offer, starting at six months, and is a great source of calcium and vitamin D. Yogurt and cheese are fermented, so the harder-to-digest proteins in milk are partially broken down, making them easier for baby to tolerate and digest. Dairy milk should be completely avoided as a beverage before age one, but it's perfectly fine to incorporate it in small amounts in meals.[6]

Myth 9: You Need to Wait Three Days Before Introducing a New Food to Your Baby

There is no evidence to support the need to wait any number of days between introducing foods. The common "three to five days rule" is outdated advice; studies actually have shown the numerous benefits of introducing new foods at a quicker pace![7] Babies need to be exposed to a large number of flavors and textures to learn the skills required to eat them. (The prime period for this is between six to twelve months old.) If you are limiting new foods to every three to five days, your baby will miss out on exposure to so many foods. You can offer your baby several different foods during a meal and don't have to limit a new food to one single option.

If you are worried about allergic reactions, most will occur within minutes to hours following exposure, not days later. The exception to this is the top nine allergens, which should be introduced one at a time to monitor for potential allergies (see page 20).

Myth 10: You Should Wait to Introduce Top Allergens Until After Age One

Current research indicates that introducing allergens early and often may lead to a reduced risk of developing food-related allergies later in life.[8] The AAP supports introducing allergens when babies begin complementary foods around six months of age.[9] Early and regular exposure to these foods may help reduce the risk that the child will develop food allergies, but if you have a family history of serious food allergies or food sensitivities, talk to your pediatrician before introducing allergens.

Myth 11: Babies Shouldn't Have Any Salt Before Age One

It is true that babies do not need added salt in their diets, but they do need some salt. Up until twelve months of age, a baby receives enough salt from breast milk or formula alone. The CDC and NHS recommend that added salt be avoided until age one, but this can be really difficult, especially because so many common items contain added salt. It's okay to offer items with added salt in moderation, but there are several ways to season foods for babies while limiting salt intake. Common foods like bread and cheese contain salt, but that doesn't mean we can't offer these items to our babies. I believe in offering certain items in moderation, and don't stress if an item contains a little added salt. When considering foods for your little one, look for options that are low in overall sodium content. The following table outlines the NHS's current recommendations for the amount of salt to give to your baby based on age.

Recommended Daily Salt Intake[10]	
Age	Salt Intake
Birth to 1 year	Less than 1 gram (400 mg), mostly received through breast milk or formula
1 to 3 years	No more than 2 grams (800 mg)
4 to 6 years	No more than 3 grams (1,200 mg)

If you are offering a food to your baby that has a higher salt content, it's a good idea to pair it with unsalted items and offer other unsalted items throughout the day to balance out their salt intake.

Myth 12: You Can't Combine Purees with Finger Foods When Doing Baby-Led Weaning

Baby-led weaning is exactly what the name says ... baby-led weaning! It doesn't matter what foods you serve or how you serve them, as long as your baby is self-feeding. We eat blended textures as adults—yogurt, applesauce, mashed potatoes, and dips, for example—and our babies can enjoy and explore these textures, too! You can offer purees on a slice of bread or on a preloaded spoon to enable self-feeding. Learning how to chew does not take away your baby's ability to swallow purees and liquids. Most babies do not have an issue switching between purees and finger foods.

Myth 13: Babies with Developmental Delays Cannot Do Baby-Led Weaning

Babies who were born prematurely or with developmental delays may have trouble self-feeding at an early age, and I advise speaking with your doctor if you have specific questions, but there are some strategies you can try if you'd like to use this feeding approach with your little one. The adapted baby-led weaning (ABLW) approach is a method for facilitating self-feeding in babies with feeding challenges. Jill Rabin, pioneer of ABLW, shares her insight on this myth: "Parents are often discouraged from attempting baby-led weaning if their child has a diagnosis such as Down syndrome or any type of feeding challenge. With ABLW, babies with feeding obstacles can safely transition to solid foods with a baby-led approach with the right guidance. The use of devices, such as a silicone feeder, may be necessary at first, but with appropriate therapeutic support, these babies can learn to self-feed a large variety of differently sized, shaped, and textured table foods."[11] Parents of children with developmental delays or feeding challenges should seek out Jill Rabin's book *Your Baby Can Self-Feed, Too* as a helpful resource on the ABLW method.

Myth 14: Introducing Fruits First Will Cause a Baby to Prefer Sweets

You may often hear people say, "Don't offer your baby fruits before vegetables, or they'll prefer sweets and not want to eat vegetables." The reality is that babies are born with an innate preference for sweet foods, whether you introduce fruits or vegetables first. According to the AAP, there's no evidence that your baby will dislike vegetables if you give them fruit first.[12] It's less about the order in which the foods are introduced and more about the consistent exposure to a variety of foods. Offering variety among all the food groups is the most important thing to expose your little one to different tastes and textures.

Myth 15: Baby-Led Weaning Means You Have to Make Separate Foods for Your Baby and Yourself

One great benefit of BLW is that your baby can eat what you eat! No need to create separate meals just for baby. Foods do need to be served and cut appropriately, and certain items need to be avoided, but your little one can enjoy all the same meals you prepare as a family, and that's what I'll teach you how to do in this book! My goal for this book is for you to be able to prepare simple recipes for your little ones that the whole family will enjoy.

I hope that this section helps clarify some common misconceptions about BLW and introducing solids. It can be information overload out there, so hopefully this will ease your mind a bit as you begin your feeding journey with your little one. And remember, I'm here to support you, no matter what feeding approach you choose!

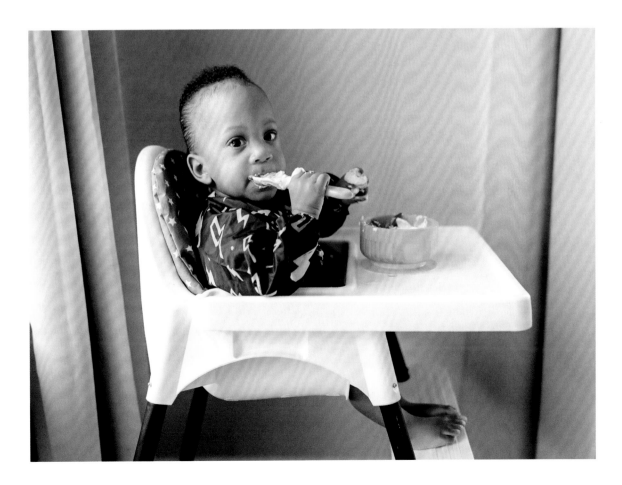

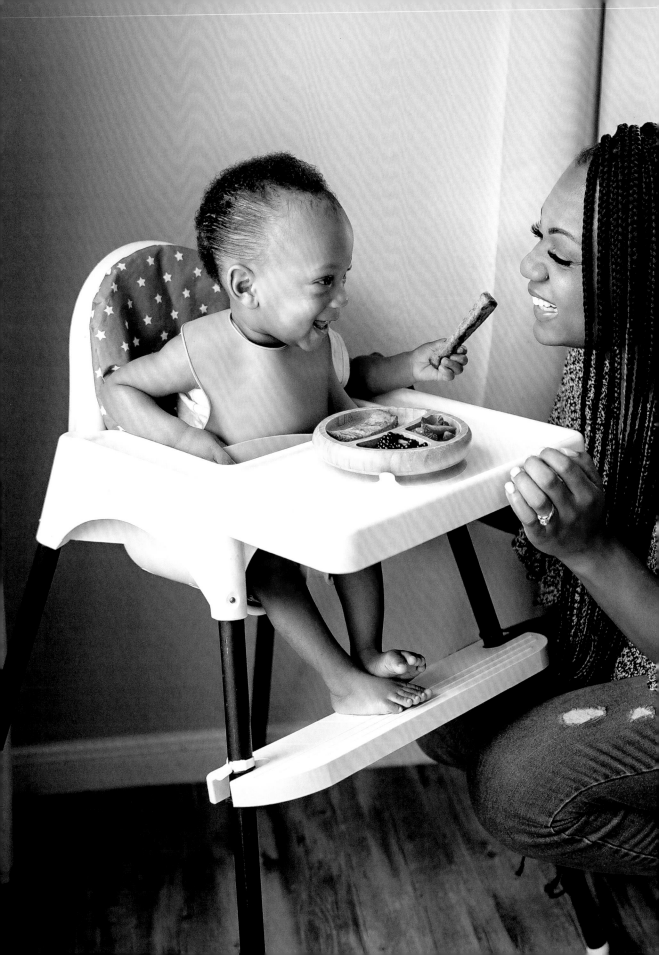

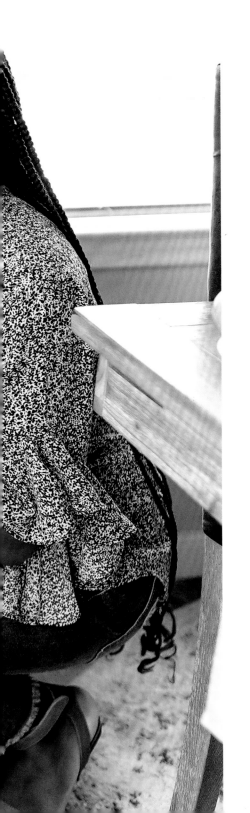

Baby-Led Weaning Resources

We've discovered what baby-led weaning is and learned how to safely prepare foods appropriate for our little ones, but what happens when things aren't so fun and dandy? What if your baby goes through a phase of throwing food on the floor? What should you do if your toddler's eating habits begin to change significantly? How do you keep your little ones busy and occupied while you're doing your best to get a meal on the table in the quickest, most stress-free way possible?

This chapter covers it all: First, I walk you through some common phases babies and toddlers often go through in their feeding journeys. Then, I share some of my favorite time-saving meal-prep tips to make feeding your family as simple as possible. I offer tips for keeping little ones busy as you cook and share some pointers for how to involve them in the kitchen. I hope that these resources are helpful as you navigate the ups and downs that come with feeding little ones!

Common Phases of Eating

Feeding little ones can definitely come with challenges, and it sometimes might feel like a roller coaster of different stages. Let's look at how to overcome some of the issues that may come up along the way.

Starting Solids: "The Beginning Phase"

Many parents are excited to start offering solid foods to their little ones, only to find that their baby has no interest in consuming these foods. The same baby who closely watched you eat different foods and always seemed to want a bite may show no desire to eat when food is placed in front of them. When you start introducing solids, your baby likely will simply play with the food. This is normal! Beginning solids is a brand-new experience for them, so don't be discouraged if your little one just plays with their food and doesn't actually eat it. Exposure to and playing with food are beneficial parts of the process. Continue offering and modeling how to eat for them.

When they do begin to taste the food, their facial expressions may seem surprising. They may make funny faces of disgust, but it doesn't necessarily mean they don't like a particular food. Continue to offer different foods and allow your baby to adjust to the new experience.

"The Food-Dropping Phase"

Ah, the dreaded food-dropping stage. You prepare what you think is your baby's favorite meal, serve it to them, and they proceed to drop every single item over the edge of the high chair tray and laugh as it hits the floor. It's frustrating, and it hurts to think about the food waste, but it's a normal part of the exploration process. What should you do if your baby is currently going through this stage?

Why Your Baby Is Dropping Food

Before we get into what to do if your baby is dropping food, let's talk about some possible reasons why they may be doing so.

- **They're discovering gravity:** Babies are learning something new every day and are fascinated by the cause-and-effect relationship. Throwing food and then seeing and hearing it drop to the floor as a result is interesting for them! They may want to eat the food but are more curious to explore.

- **They don't like it:** Your baby won't like everything you make, and that's okay! Don't let that discourage you from consistently offering that food. Sometimes, it can take multiple attempts at offering a food item before a baby decides to give it a try.

- **They want to get out of their chair:** Sometimes, babies begin to throw food on the floor to indicate that they're finished eating. They may also be bored with sitting in a chair, or they might be tired, so throwing food is their way of communicating that they want out. They may also simply not be hungry.

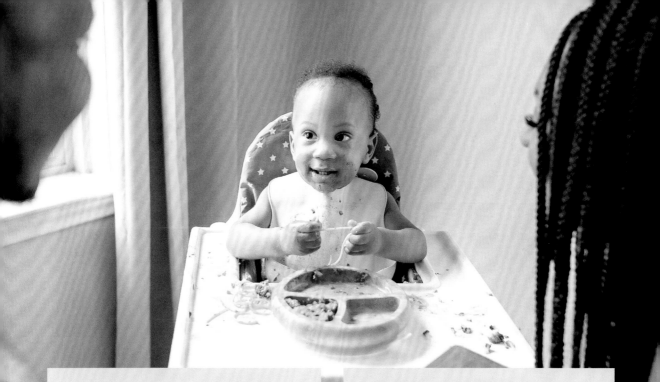

What to Do When Baby Drops Food on the Floor

Sometimes, food ends up on the floor by mistake, but at other times, it's definitely intentional. Here are some suggestions to dealing with food-dropping:

- **Don't react:** This is easier said than done, but if your baby is purposely dropping food on the floor, try not to react. Babies are so smart and can sense our energy. They love the chance to get a big reaction out of us, and seeing a big reaction may lead to them reattempting the behavior to keep getting that reaction. Calmly remind them that food stays on the table.

- **Eat with your baby:** Try your best to share all meals with your baby. Babies want your attention and may drop food on the floor in hopes of getting it, so sitting with them and sharing meals with them may help prevent this.

To Replace or Not to Replace?

There are different opinions on whether you should replace the food after baby has dropped it. One view is that you shouldn't, so baby gets the message that once the food is dropped, it's gone for good. Another perspective is to repeatedly replace the food in case baby is still hungry but was just exploring how gravity works. Try to find a middle ground between these two options by replacing the food one or two times. Your baby may still be hungry, so try offering another serving to see if they will eat it. If your baby continues to drop the food, it may just be time to end the meal.

Remember, this is okay! It's likely just a phase as your baby continues to grow and become more aware of their surroundings. Dropping food is a normal part of the process of learning cause and effect. Babies are exploring and learning new things every day, so if you're also going through the food-dropping stage, just keep in mind that, as with many things, this is just a phase! Be patient and it will pass.

"The Barely Eating Phase"

It's so easy to feel discouraged when our babies don't eat well. We immediately jump to blaming ourselves and assuming that we are doing something wrong. It can be tempting to try to force our little ones to eat a little more to ensure they eat "enough," but what exactly qualifies as "enough"? Oftentimes, our version of "enough" is much more than what their bodies know is enough. So what should we do if our babies barely eat a meal?

- **Let them be:** Babies are in tune with their bodies and know when they want to eat. With baby-led weaning (BLW), it's difficult to measure how much a baby eats. With purees, we can physically see an amount in a container, but with BLW, a good amount of food may end up in other places. Seeing food all over the floor and high chair may make us think that our babies didn't eat a thing, but they often consume more than we think.

- **Don't try to force-feed:** This can have many negative effects down the line, like causing your child to form negative associations with food. One benefit of BLW is that babies are in control of their food intake, so try to continue to offer that sense of independence.

- **Don't be discouraged:** I know, this is a hard one. It can be so upsetting when we prepare a meal that our baby barely eats. But even if baby just tastes the foods, they'll be getting some nutrients.

- **Try again at the next meal:** Remember the division of responsibility: Our job as caregivers is to offer meals; it is baby's job to decide what and how much to eat.

- **Keep offering milk:** Always remember that breast milk and/or formula should always be a baby's primary source of nutrition until age one.

Factors That Can Affect How a Baby Eats

Many factors could affect how a baby eats at a particular time. Being mindful of these factors helps put our minds at ease if our babies are not eating as much as we would like:

- **Lack of appetite:** This one may seem obvious, but many times when a baby doesn't eat, it's simply because they just are not hungry. A baby may have filled up with milk or other meals beforehand, so it's normal for them to not be hungry during a particular meal.

- **Tiredness:** No one wants to eat when they're sleepy. If baby is overtired, they will not have the energy to to eat.

- **Discomfort:** Babies should be in a comfortable seated position while eating. Be sure that they are seated appropriately and that their high chair seat belt is comfortably tightened.

- **Being overwhelmed:** There are so many things that can overwhelm and distract a baby while eating. Anything from having too much food on the table to too much background noise can be overstimulating. Try to make mealtimes a calm, relaxing experience by offering smaller portions and decreasing noise as much as possible.

- **Illness:** Illnesses affect how we adults eat, and the same goes for babies. It is normal for their appetites to decrease if they are battling an illness.

- **Time of day:** It's common for a baby to eat more in the morning and less as the day goes on. Even we, as adults, may not have the best appetites in the evenings if we eat larger meals during the day.

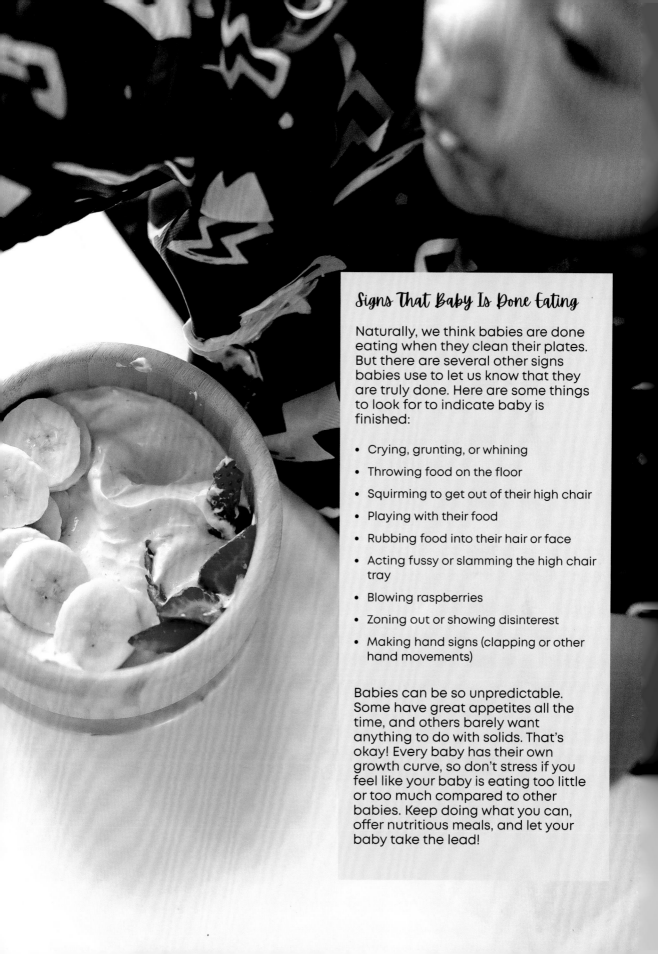

Signs That Baby Is Done Eating

Naturally, we think babies are done eating when they clean their plates. But there are several other signs babies use to let us know that they are truly done. Here are some things to look for to indicate baby is finished:

- Crying, grunting, or whining
- Throwing food on the floor
- Squirming to get out of their high chair
- Playing with their food
- Rubbing food into their hair or face
- Acting fussy or slamming the high chair tray
- Blowing raspberries
- Zoning out or showing disinterest
- Making hand signs (clapping or other hand movements)

Babies can be so unpredictable. Some have great appetites all the time, and others barely want anything to do with solids. That's okay! Every baby has their own growth curve, so don't stress if you feel like your baby is eating too little or too much compared to other babies. Keep doing what you can, offer nutritious meals, and let your baby take the lead!

"The Fussy Toddler Phase"

Do you have a toddler who was a great eater as a baby but is now eating significantly less? This may seem strange, but it's actually a very common phase many toddlers go through.

My Toddler Isn't Interested in Eating

If your toddler doesn't seem keen on eating, keep the following in mind:

- As toddlers are growing physically, their minds are growing at a constant rate as well. Toddlers are so interested in everything around them, and sitting down to eat a meal is probably at the bottom of the list of things they'd like to explore.

- Try to set some mealtime structures so that there are clear expectations in place for mealtime, but allow toddlers to take control of what and how much to eat.

- Know that picky eating is normal. Toddlers begin to develop preferences and go through phases of loving and not loving certain foods.

Why Is My Toddler Eating Much Less?

Toddlers eat less for a variety of reasons:

- Between the ages of one and five, it's completely normal for a toddler's appetite to diminish. After all, toddlers don't grow as fast as babies do.

- Think about how much growth a baby goes through from the newborn stage to age one. Most full-term babies double their birth weight by six months of age and triple it by the time they are a year old. Plus, consider how quickly you went through size newborn, size 1, and size 2 diapers. Then, it feels like they're in size 3 and size 4 diapers forever!

- When they hit toddlerhood, the growth spurts slow down. They gain weight much less quickly, resulting in decreased appetites.

- You may feel like your toddler isn't eating enough or is never hungry, but they are matching their growth rate.

Making Mealtimes Enjoyable

Here are some tips for getting through mealtimes with fussy eaters:

- Don't force-feed. Force-feeding can have negative effects on your baby and can cause them to develop a poor relationship with food down the line.

- Don't leave your child sitting at the table alone to finish their meal after everyone else is done eating. This makes them feel excluded.

- Don't make a big deal to your child about how little or how much they eat. Mealtimes should be an enjoyable experience, and making a big deal if they finish their plate or if they're not eating much brings unneeded pressure to the table.

- Don't threaten them or bargain with them. This will only drive you away from the goal of setting healthy relationships with food and may result in a constant power struggle instead. Continue to offer a variety of foods, and try to make things interesting and fun. Involve your toddler in the kitchen, and work to make mealtimes an enjoyable experience for all.

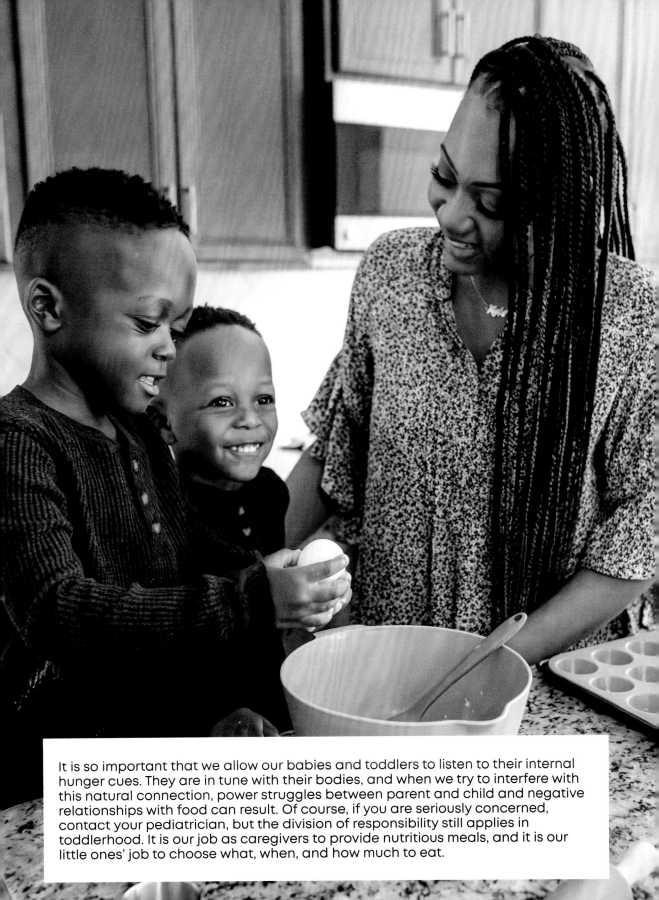

It is so important that we allow our babies and toddlers to listen to their internal hunger cues. They are in tune with their bodies, and when we try to interfere with this natural connection, power struggles between parent and child and negative relationships with food can result. Of course, if you are seriously concerned, contact your pediatrician, but the division of responsibility still applies in toddlerhood. It is our job as caregivers to provide nutritious meals, and it is our little ones' job to choose what, when, and how much to eat.

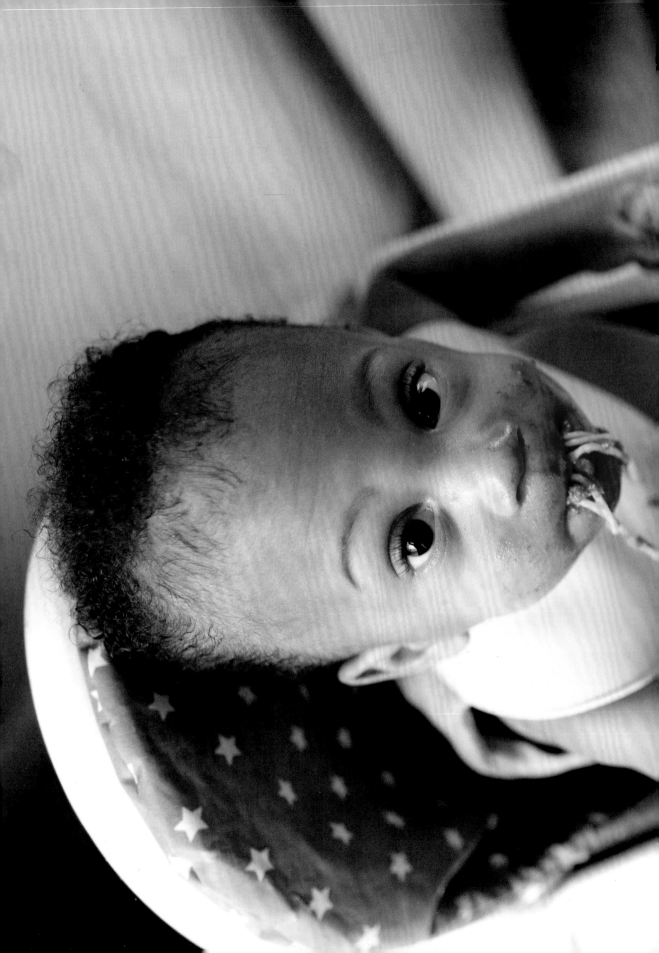

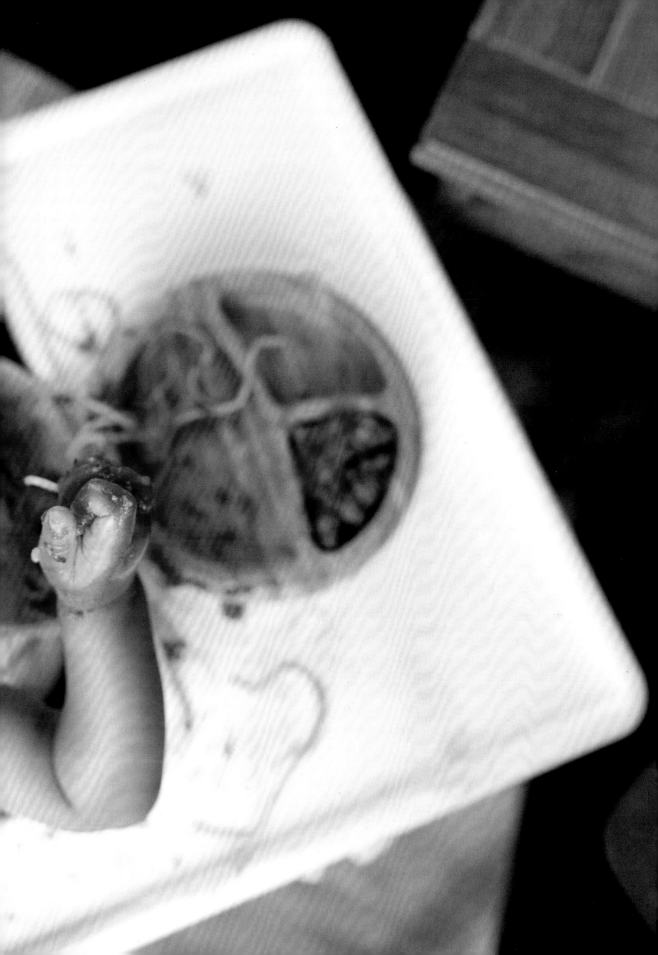

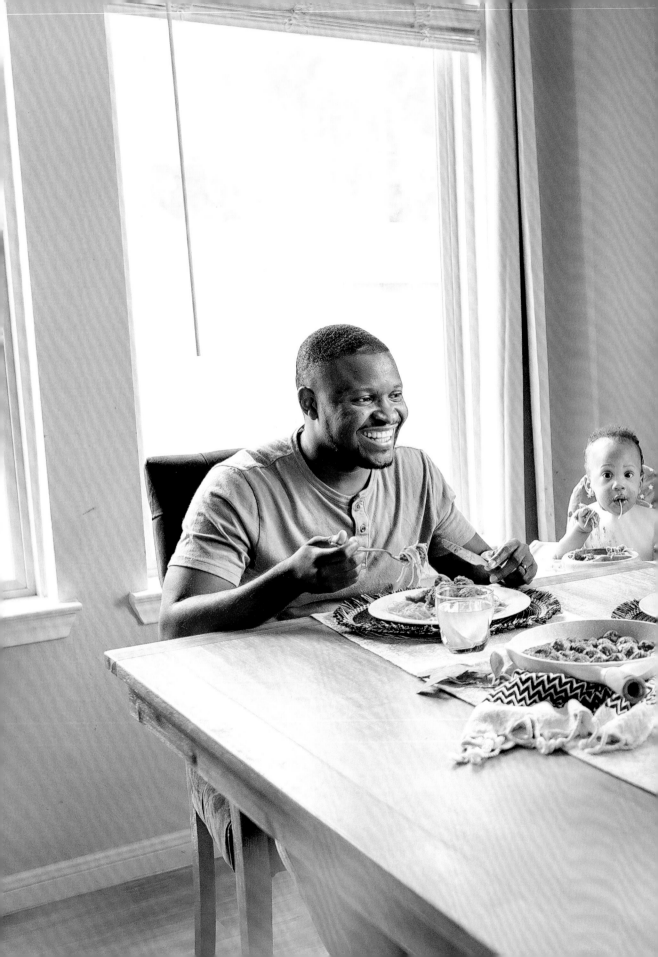

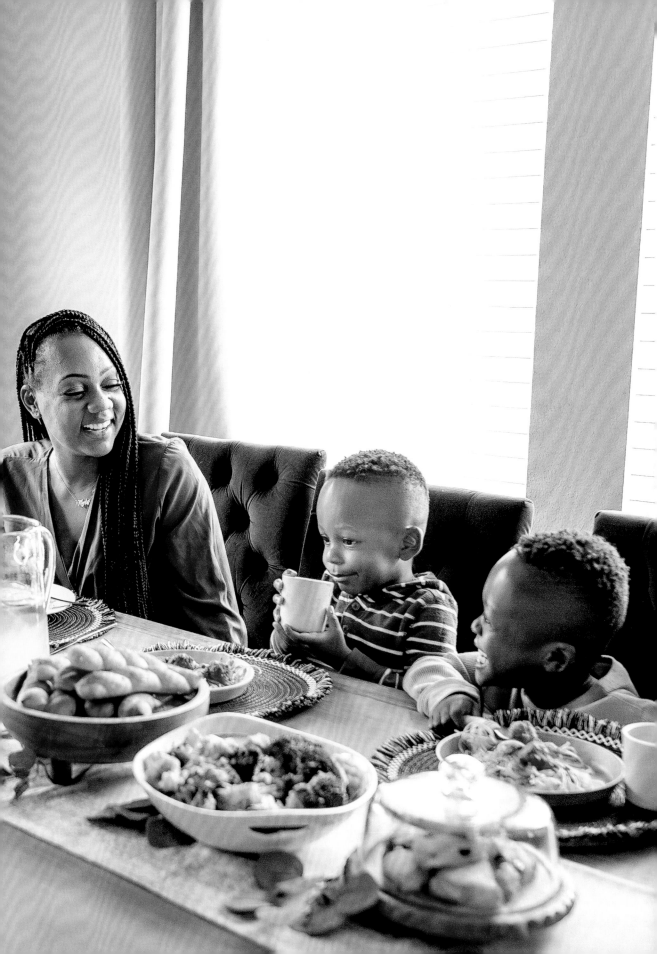

Sample Meal Plan & Grocery List

The following section contains a sample meal plan and accompanying grocery list. This meal plan is a guide to help keep you organized and give you structure for planning meals throughout a week. I've also included my top time-saving tips for meal prepping as well as tips and tricks for cooking with little ones.

Meal Planning

Meal planning can be a great way to organize meals for your little ones to serve throughout the week. Meal planning isn't for everyone, but charting out what to feed baby for the week can help us feel a little more organized and less stressed as parents. Of course, meal plans don't have to be set in stone, as plans change and life happens, but it is nice to have an idea of what meals you'd like to serve and what groceries are needed for those meals. To help with meal planning, I've put together a sample meal plan with an accompanying grocery list for a week of meals that the whole family can enjoy!

Sample One-Week Meal Plan			
Day	Breakfast	Lunch	Dinner
Sunday	Berry Smoothie Bowl (page 65)	Spinach & Tomato Quesadillas (page 130)	Veggie-Packed Beef Meatballs (page 160) with spaghetti
Monday	Banana Overnight Oats (page 74), prepped on Sunday	Sweet Potato Chicken Nuggets (page 121), prepped on Sunday	Meatball subs with leftover Veggie-Packed Beef Meatballs (page 160)
Tuesday	Broccoli & Cheese Egg Bites (page 77), prepped on Sunday, with fruit	Peanut Butter Banana "Sushi" Rolls (page 137)	Taco Chili (page 175)
Wednesday	Buttered toast, fruit, and yogurt	Spinach & Tomato Quesadillas (page 130)	Leftover Taco Chili (page 175), served over rice
Thursday	Banana Overnight Oats (page 74)	Avocado toast (mash ½ of an avocado on a slice of toast)	Stuffed Shells Bake (page 164)
Friday	Broccoli & Cheese Egg Bites (page 77) with fruit	Strawberry Cheesecake "Sushi" Rolls (page 137)	Leftover Stuffed Shells Bake (page 164)
Saturday	Blackberry Cheesecake French Toast Sticks (page 70)	Sweet Potato Chicken Nuggets (page 121)	Order takeout!

Grocery List

After I fill in my meal plan with ideas for what I'd like to make throughout the week, I put together a grocery list of items I'll need for each recipe. I check off items that I already have in my fridge or pantry and limit the list to only the items I need. Doing this helps me focus on only what is needed when grocery shopping because it is so easy to get carried away and overspend otherwise.

Sample Weekly Grocery List					
Proteins	**Dairy**	**Grains**	**Fruits**	**Vegetables**	**Pantry Items**
Chicken breast	Butter (unsalted)	Bread rolls	Avocados	Beets (cooked)	Coconut milk
Eggs	Cream cheese	Granola	Bananas	Broccoli	Maple syrup
Ground chicken	Greek yogurt	Jumbo shell pasta	Blackberries	Canned beans (black and kidney)	Marinara sauce
Ground beef	Heavy cream	Panko breadcrumbs	Blueberries	Canned corn	Natural peanut butter
	Milk	Spaghetti	Strawberries	Canned diced tomatoes	Oil (mild-tasting)
	Parmesan	Rolled oats	Frozen mixed berries	Carrots	Tomato sauce
	Ricotta	Rice		Onions	
	Shredded cheese (cheddar and mozzarella)	Sandwich bread		Spinach	
	Sour cream	Tortillas		Sweet potatoes	
				Roma tomatoes	
				Zucchini	

Time-Saving Meal Prep Tips

If you're like me, you're a busy parent trying to get good, nutritious food on the table but don't want to spend all day or night in the kitchen. Here are some tips to help:

- **Meal plan:** Meal planning is a great way to save time when preparing meals. Knowing exactly what you're going to make each day takes the guesswork out of trying to figure out meals and ingredients on the spot, ultimately saving time in the kitchen.

- **Meal prep:** Once you know what you'll make, take some time to prepare any ingredients that you can. Chopping up foods and portioning out ingredients ahead of time may seem like small tasks but can save you so much time. You'll thank yourself later for prepping items!

- **Use frozen and canned foods:** Having prepackaged food items on hand is great for putting together a quick meal. I love taking basic canned or jarred foods and jazzing them up with other flavors. Frozen fruits and vegetables are great to have around and are just as nutritious as fresh.

- **Cook in bulk:** Making foods in advance and freezing them to use throughout the week helps make mealtimes much more manageable. Breakfast can be especially tricky during busy mornings, so having a freezer stash of items to quickly grab and reheat is a game changer. You can prep meals the weekend before, freeze them, and quickly reheat them when needed to serve.

- **Repurpose leftovers**: Use leftovers to your advantage! Make extra servings of meals with the intention of using the leftovers for another meal the next day. I know that leftovers aren't everyone's cup of tea, but do they really count as leftovers if you incorporate them into another meal in a creative way?

Tips for Cooking with Kids

Finding time to cook meals for the family is one thing, but managing cooking while having a fussy baby at your hip or a toddler pulling at your leg is a whole other ball game. Here are some tips to help make cooking with kids a little easier.

Keeping Little Ones Busy

Providing your little ones with tasks and activities while you cook helps keep them busy and entertained and gives you a few undisturbed minutes to put a meal together. Here are some of my favorite ways to keep little ones entertained while preparing a meal.

For Babies

- **Teething toys:** Teething toys are great for babies to gnaw on to soothe their little gums.

- **Black-and-white books or toys:** Babies love the contrast of black and white, so having high-contrast books and toys can help hold their attention for a few minutes.

- **Mirrors:** Try popping a mirror in front of your little one while you work. It can spark their curiosity and encourage them to hold up their head!

- **Bouncer seat or playmat:** Having a designated place to lay down your baby is extremely helpful so that you can have your hands free to prepare a meal. Bouncer seats and playmats are great options to help keep your little one self-entertained and occupied for a few minutes.

- **Baby wrap or carrier:** Some babies love to be held, so using a wrap or carrier gives you the ability to keep baby close while still having your hands free to prep foods.

For Toddlers

- **Coloring books:** Give your little one a few crayons or markers and coloring pages, and let them have fun scribbling all over the page. You can also give them large blank sheets and let them go at it!

- **Play-Doh:** This is great for toddlers over the age of three. Give your little one some cookie cutters and Play-Doh, and let them use their creativity to come up with different creations.

- **Tiles and blocks:** Tiles and blocks are great tools for little ones to work on coordination and balance skills. They can enjoy the process of building, breaking, and repeating.

- **Magnets:** Magnets come in all different shapes, sizes, and styles—from alphabet letters to animals. Let them have fun sticking different magnets on the fridge as you prep meals.

- **Music:** You can never go wrong with a mini dance party! Play some music and let your little one sing and dance with a pretend mic.

- **FaceTime:** Allowing your little one to enjoy a video call with a family member is a great way to keep them occupied while staying in touch with family, especially if you live far away.

- **Kitchen play:** Plastic storage containers, spatulas, and mixing bowls can go a long way when it comes to entertaining kids. Something about the aspect of playing with "real items" always seems more fun than playing with toys. Plus, you can keep an eye on your little one in the kitchen as you prepare meal items.

Involving Your Little Ones in the Kitchen

When your little one is old enough to take on small tasks, try getting them involved in the kitchen with you! This will be a great bonding experience and has so many benefits: It can encourage independence, promote number sense, and potentially prevent picky eating. Cooking with kids also comes with some challenges, so here are some tips to help make the process a little easier:

- **Pick a good time:** Timing is so important when it comes to doing any activity with kids. You wouldn't want to take your child on a trip to the zoo when they're sleepy and cranky. The same applies to being in the kitchen. Cook together when your child is well rested and happy. Trying to cook with a child who is cranky, hungry, or tired probably won't be fun, so be sure the time is right.

- **Plan ahead:** Get as many ingredients ready ahead of time as you can, before you get started with your child. If a recipe calls for room-temperature butter or eggs, take those out beforehand. Premeasure ingredients and have them laid out on the counter and ready to go. Kids are notoriously impatient and likely won't want to wait for you to gather ingredients to measure while they are waiting to move on to the next task. Kids also love to dump things, so premeasuring ensures that the recipe still turns out as planned with less room for error. I learned this lesson the hard way the first time I baked with my son. I asked him to pour a tiny amount of vanilla extract into some cupcake batter. My definition of "a little" was a small splash, but my son's definition was the entire bottle. Needless to say, those cupcakes were packed with vanilla flavor!

- **Embrace the mess:** Cooking and baking with kids will definitely result in a mess. It's inevitable. Be prepared to have flour all over the counter (and potentially the floor, your child, yourself, and your pets), eggshells mixed into the batter, and sprinkles in your child's hair at the end of the day. Messes happen, but they are okay! Have towels and cleaning cloths on hand to make the cleanup easier. Involve your little ones in the cleanup process, too, so you're not left to deal with a huge mess alone at the end and so your little ones can practice cleaning up after themselves.

- **Be safe:** This one is a given, but be sure your little one is safe throughout the cooking process. Give them age-appropriate tasks, and take charge of any steps that may put your little one at risk of getting cut or burned. If you would like your little one to do any cutting, use child-safe tools so that they can be involved in a safe way. We don't want our little ones getting hurt!

- **Be patient:** This is easier said than done. It's easy to lose our patience when our little ones get impatient, want to take charge of certain steps, and get frustrated when they can't do something, but losing our patience and getting upset will only make the experience tense and unenjoyable. Try to let go of the idea of perfection when cooking and baking with your little one. It's okay if the cookies aren't decorated perfectly. It's okay if your child accidentally drops an egg on the floor. Try to take a breath, remain calm, and laugh at the messy moments. There may be frustrating parts throughout the process, but try to think about the joy your little one will have bonding with you through cooking.

Cooking while tending to little ones can be a challenging task, but try to savor this time when they're still little. Despite these stressful moments, you'll make memories that you'll cherish forever. I hope that these tips will help make getting meals on the table a little more manageable.

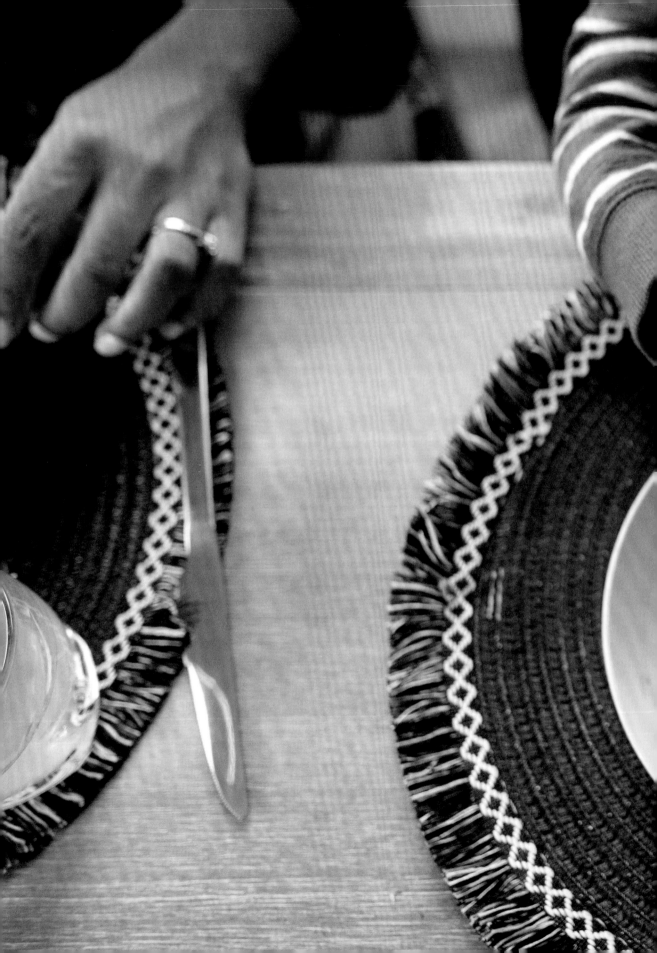

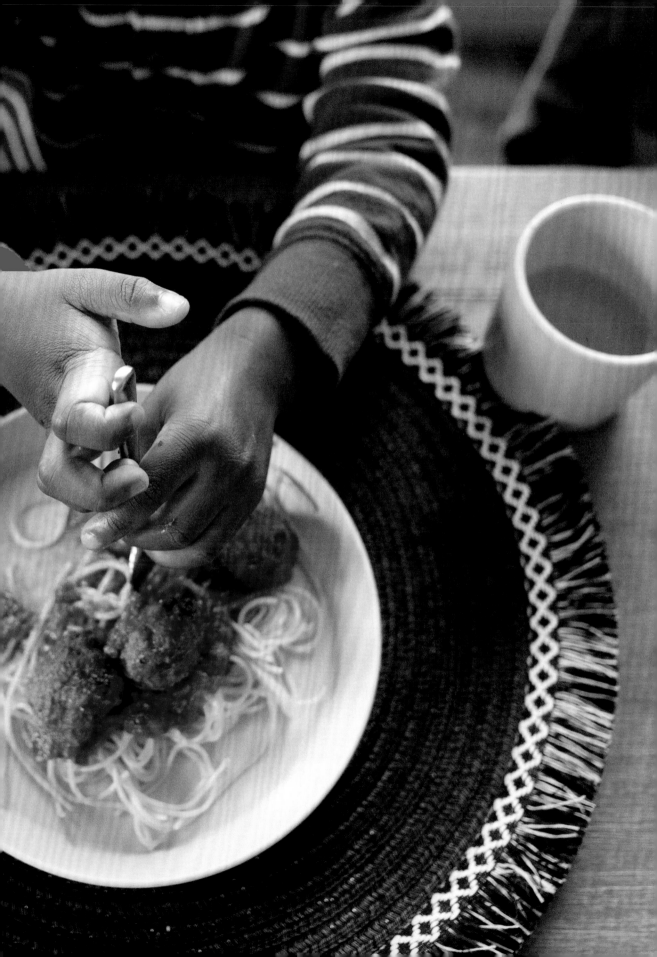

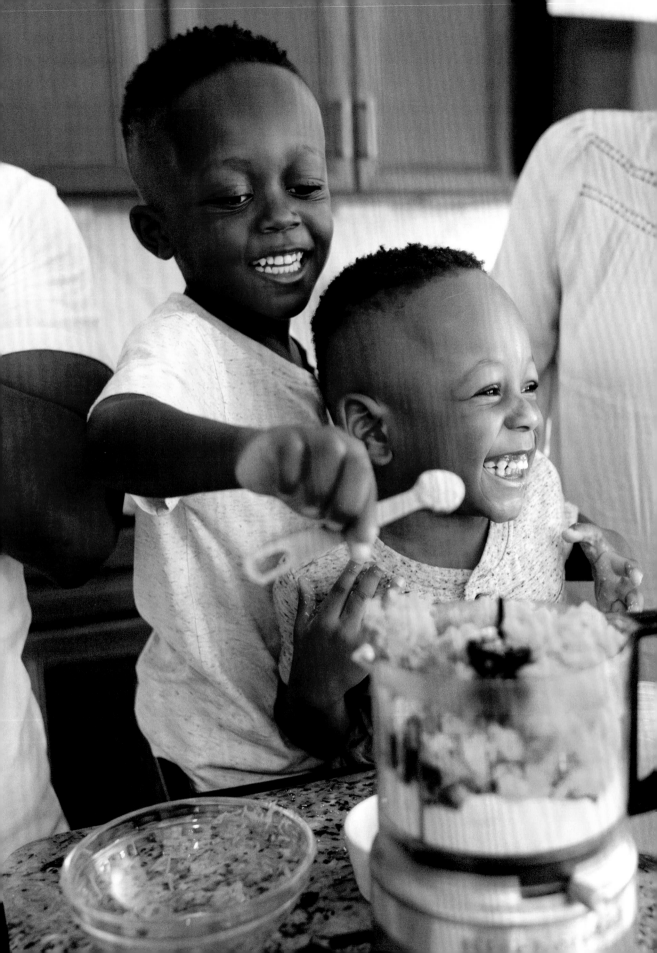

Recipe Guide

Every recipe in this book was created with the busy parent in mind, so each requires a minimal amount of time to prepare and calls for common ingredients. My hope is that many of the ingredients are items you already have on hand or are easily accessible in your local grocery store.

As you get cooking, you'll notice a few symbols by many of the recipes. Each recipe is labeled with the following dietary icons, as appropriate, so that you know at a glance which recipes are suitable for your family. I've also suggested ingredient substitutions for common allergenic foods when possible.

DF • **Made without dairy.**

EF • **Made without eggs.**

GF • **Made without wheat or other gluten-containing ingredients. (To ensure that a recipe that calls for oats is gluten-free, use certified gluten-free rolled oats.).**

NF • **Made without peanuts or tree nuts.**

V • **Meat- and fish-free; suitable for vegetarians. (May contain eggs.)**

Salt is listed as an optional ingredient in some recipes and can be omitted, if desired. In many cases, you can remove your baby's portion of the dish and add salt to the remaining dish for the rest of the family.

Maple syrup can be omitted or replaced with a natural fruit sweetener as necessary.

"Mild-tasting oil" is called for in some recipes and refers to those oils that have neutral flavor. Examples include avocado oil, coconut oil, and extra-light-tasting olive oils. These oils ensure that the food won't have a strong oily taste.

In some recipes, an egg can be substituted with a "flax egg." To make a flax egg, combine 3 tablespoons of water with 1 tablespoon of ground flaxseed. Let the mixture sit in the fridge for about 15 minutes or until it forms a gel.

Now, if you're ready to start creating some simple and nutritious recipes for your tiny bellies and the whole family, let's dive in!

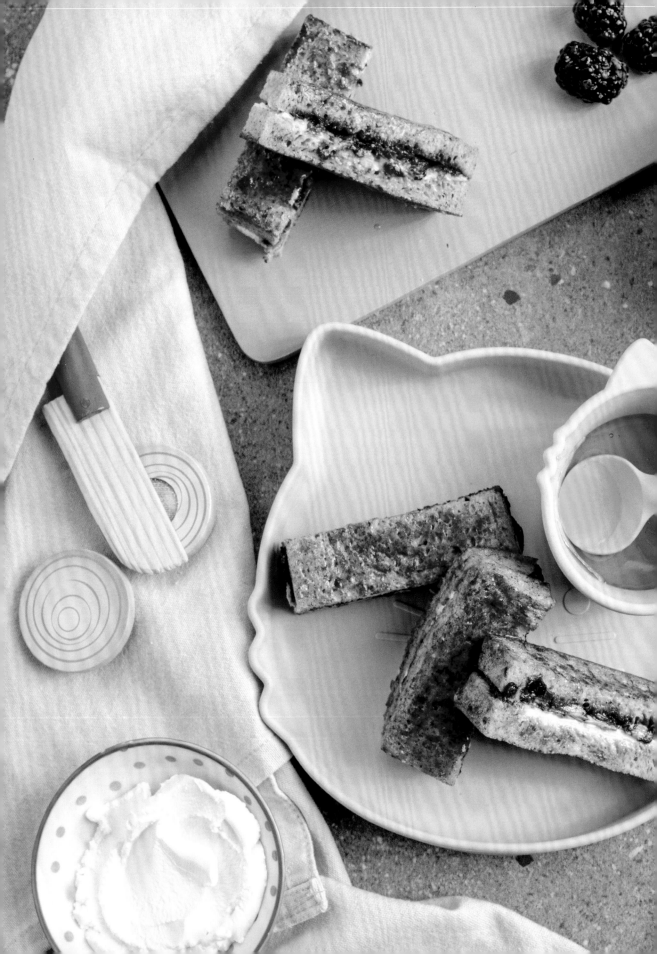

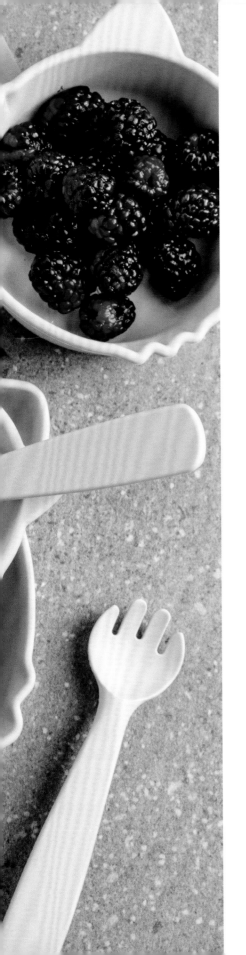

Breakfast

They say "Breakfast is the most important meal of the day" for a reason. Breakfast is vital for nourishing our bodies first thing in the morning, and it's no different for our little ones. After a long night of sleep, you may find that your baby has a great appetite in the morning and is ready for their morning meal. Start the day with these simple, filling breakfast recipes, and you and your little one will be fueled and ready for the day!

Sweet Potato Muffins

prep **8 minutes** / cook **15 minutes** / makes **18 mini muffins**

½ cup (120 g) mashed cooked sweet potato (see Tip 1)

1 egg (see Tip 2)

3 tablespoons mild-tasting oil

2 tablespoons unsweetened applesauce

2 tablespoons maple syrup

½ cup (45 g) old-fashioned rolled oats

½ cup (65 g) all-purpose flour

1 teaspoon baking powder

1 teaspoon ground cinnamon

Sweet potato is such a versatile vegetable, wonderful in both savory and sweet dishes, and it adds the perfect amount of sweetness to these mini muffins. They are soft and fluffy with some added texture from the rolled oats. Everything comes together in one bowl, and they will have your home smelling like warm cinnamon and spices as they bake!

1 Preheat the oven to 350°F (180°C).

2 Whisk together the sweet potato, egg, oil, applesauce, and maple syrup in a large bowl until smooth.

3 Add the oats, flour, baking powder, and cinnamon, and mix until just combined.

4 Scoop tablespoon-sized portions of batter into a 24-cup silicone mini-muffin pan (see Tip 3).

5 Bake for 15 minutes, or until a knife inserted into the center of a muffin comes out clean. Let cool completely before serving.

Storage

Store in an airtight container at room temperature for up to 2 days or in the fridge for up to 5 days. To freeze, store in a freezer-safe bag with most of the air removed for up to 3 months. To reheat, microwave for 30 seconds, or until warmed through. You can also thaw completely at room temperature.

Tips

1. You may precook the sweet potato in the oven (poke holes in the potato, and bake at 425°F/220°C for 45 to 50 minutes, until tender) or in the microwave (poke holes in the potato, and microwave for 5 or 6 minutes, until tender). When the potato is fully cooled, peel and mash it.

2. Egg-free? Swap the egg with a flax egg (see page 55).

3. If you don't have a silicone mini-muffin pan, you can use a metal 24-cup mini-muffin pan. If using a metal mini-muffin pan, be sure to grease the pan with cooking spray or butter so the muffins won't stick.

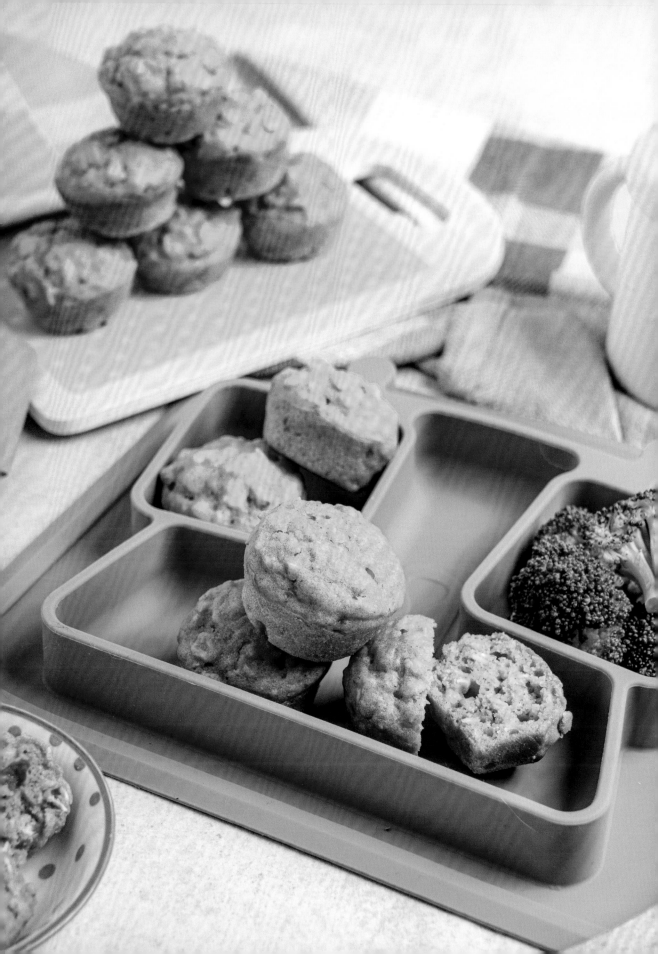

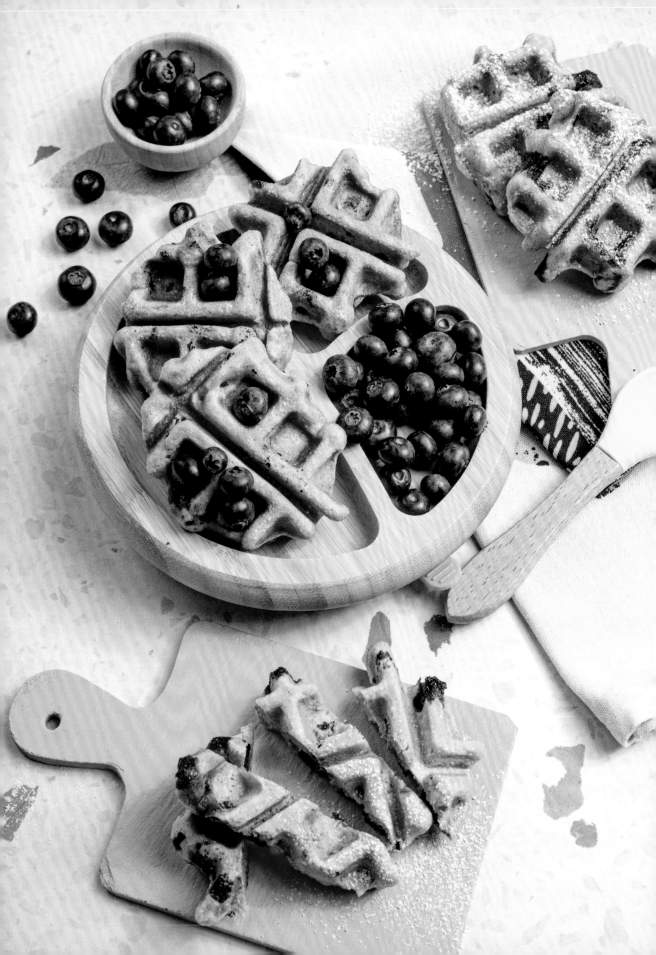

Blueberry Banana Waffles

prep **5 minutes** / cook **10 minutes** / makes **10 mini waffles**

Cooking spray (olive or avocado oil)

1 large overripe banana

1 cup (90 g) old-fashioned rolled oats

2 eggs (see Tip 1)

2 tablespoons mild-tasting oil

1 teaspoon baking powder

½ teaspoon ground cinnamon

¼ teaspoon vanilla extract

⅓ cup (50 g) blueberries (see Tip 2)

Powdered sugar, for dusting (optional)

Maple syrup, for serving (optional)

These blender waffles are simple to make for a sweet morning breakfast. They are naturally sweetened with overripe bananas and blueberries and are soft textured, making them easy for little ones to break apart and eat.

1 Preheat a waffle maker. Spray the waffle maker with cooking spray to prevent sticking.

2 Blend the banana, oats, eggs, oil, baking powder, cinnamon, and vanilla extract in a blender until smooth. Stir in the blueberries.

3 Pour ¼ cup (60 ml) of batter onto the waffle maker, and cook according to your waffle maker's instructions. The waffles should be firm on the outside and golden brown when cooked. Transfer the cooked waffles to a plate, cover with a towel to keep warm, and repeat with the remaining batter.

4 Serve with powdered sugar and maple syrup if using (see Tip 3).

Storage

Store cooled waffles in an airtight container in the refrigerator for up to 2 days. To freeze, store in a freezer-safe bag with most of the air removed for up to 2 months. To reheat, microwave for 30 seconds, or until warmed through. You can also reheat them in the toaster on the lowest setting for 2 or 3 minutes, until warmed through.

Tips

1. Egg-free? Swap the eggs with a liquid egg substitute like JUST Egg.
2. When serving fresh blueberries to babies or young toddlers, quarter them or smash them into discs to eliminate roundness. Whole, uncooked blueberries are a choking hazard.
3. Serve to baby as is or with powdered sugar and maple syrup on top for the rest of the family.

DF EF GF V

Apple Pie Breakfast Bars

prep **10 minutes** / cook **20 minutes** / makes **8 bars**

½ cup (45 g) old-fashioned rolled oats

½ cup (50 g) oat flour (see Tip 1)

½ teaspoon baking powder

½ teaspoon ground cinnamon

⅓ cup (82 g) unsweetened applesauce

3 tablespoons maple syrup (optional, see Tip 2)

2 tablespoons natural peanut butter, plus more for drizzling (see Tips 3 and 4)

½ large apple (preferably Honeycrisp or Fuji)

Granola bars are a great grab-and-go breakfast option for busy mornings, but store-bought versions can get pricey. I was inspired to create a homemade bar with minimal ingredients for hurried mornings and came up with these apple oatmeal bars. They are quick to whip up and are the perfect soft-textured treat.

1 Preheat the oven to 350°F (180°C). Place a sheet of parchment paper in a 9 × 5-inch (23 × 13 cm) loaf pan and press down, allowing some of the paper to hang over the sides of the pan.

2 Combine the oats, oat flour, baking powder, and cinnamon in a large bowl.

3 Whisk together the applesauce, maple syrup, and peanut butter in a medium bowl until smooth.

4 Pour the wet ingredients into the bowl with the dry ingredients.

5 Grate the apple using a box grater, add the apple to the bowl, and mix until combined.

6 Press the mixture into the loaf pan. Use a spatula to flatten and evenly smooth out the top.

7 Bake for 20 minutes, or until the edges are golden brown.

8 Let cool completely in the pan, slice into eight bars, and serve.

Storage

Store in an airtight container at room temperature for up to 3 days. To freeze, store in a freezer-safe bag with most of the air removed for up to 3 months. To reheat, microwave for 30 seconds, or until warmed through. You can also thaw completely at room temperature.

Tips

1. To make your own oat flour, blend ½ cup (45 g) of dry old-fashioned rolled oats in a high-powered blender or a food processor until very fine.
2. If preparing these bars for a young baby, omit the maple syrup.
3. Drizzle a little peanut butter on top of the bars for some added protein and flavor.
4. Nut-free? Replace the peanut butter with a seed-based butter, or omit it completely..

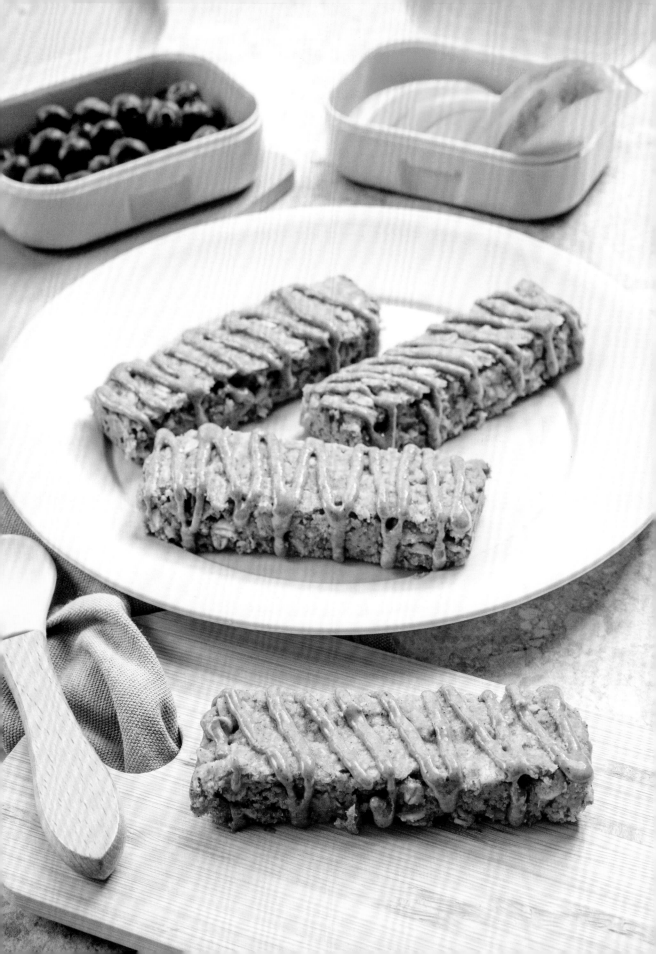

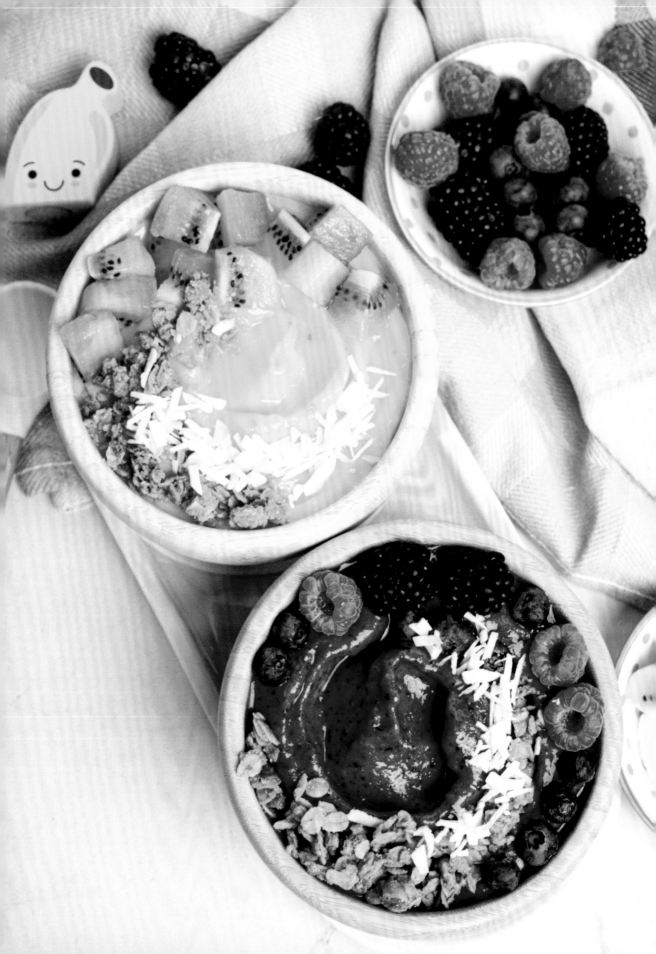

Smoothie Bowls

prep **5 minutes** / serves **1 adult & 1 child**

Tropical Smoothie Bowl

Smoothie Bowl

1 cup (150 g) frozen mango chunks

1 cup (150 g) frozen pineapple chunks

1 medium overripe banana

3 tablespoons coconut milk

Toppings

Finely crushed granola

Sliced banana

Sliced mango or pineapple

Diced kiwi

Unsweetened shredded coconut

Berry Smoothie Bowl

Smoothie Bowl

2 cups (300 g) frozen mixed berries

1 large overripe banana

3 to 4 tablespoons coconut milk

Toppings

Finely crushed granola

Mixed berries

Unsweetened shredded coconut

Smoothie bowls are a great way to serve a variety of fruits all at once. They are a refreshing breakfast treat and can be customized with your little one's favorite toppings. The tropical and mixed berry flavors are so satisfying for a fresh, naturally sweetened treat. This recipe makes enough for you and your baby to enjoy together!

1 Add all the smoothie bowl ingredients for your preferred flavor to a food processor or high-powered blender (see Tip 1), and blend until smooth, scraping down the sides as needed. The mixture will be thick, but continue blending in increments until incorporated (see Tip 2).

2 Pour the mixture into small bowls, add the toppings, and serve (see Tip 3).

Storage

Smoothie bowls are best enjoyed fresh but can be frozen for future use in an airtight container for up to 3 months and thawed. Break them up with a fork occasionally as they thaw to get a slushy, smoothie consistency.

Tips

1. Blend some hemp hearts into the mixture for some added fats and omega-3s!
2. Add extra tablespoons of milk if needed, but don't add too much; you want the mixture to be thick in consistency.
3. If topping with berries, quarter or smash them before serving.

Peanut Butter Banana Bread

prep **10 minutes** / cook **40 minutes** / makes **12 slices**

3 medium overripe bananas

½ cup (125 g) natural peanut butter (see Tip 1)

2 eggs (see Tip 2)

1¾ cups (175 g) almond flour

2 teaspoons baking powder

1 teaspoon ground cinnamon

¼ teaspoon salt (optional)

Peanut butter and banana is an unmatched combination that pairs together so well in this fluffy, moist, and delicious bread. The peanut butter adds rich flavor and helps make the bread incredibly soft. Peanut butter has always been my favorite spread, so if you're also a peanut butter lover, you'll love this bread!

1 Preheat the oven to 350°F (180°C). Line a 9 × 5-inch (23 × 13 cm) loaf pan with parchment paper.

2 Mash the bananas with a fork in a large bowl until smooth.

3 Add the peanut butter and eggs, and whisk until well incorporated.

4 Add the almond flour, baking powder, cinnamon, and salt (if using), and mix until well combined.

5 Pour the mixture into the loaf pan, and bake for 40 minutes, or until a knife inserted into the center comes out clean.

6 Let cool completely in the pan, then slice and serve.

Storage

Store in an airtight container at room temperature for up to 2 days or in the fridge for up to 5 days. To freeze, store in a freezer-safe airtight container for up to 3 months. To reheat, place on a parchment paper–lined baking sheet, and bake in 350°F (180°C) oven for 20 to 25 minutes, until warmed through. You can also let the bread thaw at room temperature for 2 or 3 hours.

Tips

1. Nut-free? Replace the peanut butter with a seed-based butter, replace the almond flour with all-purpose flour, and add ⅓ cup (80 ml) of milk. You may also want to add a little maple syrup because the batter will not be as naturally sweet without the almond flour.

2. Egg-free? Swap the eggs with a liquid egg substitute like JUST Egg.

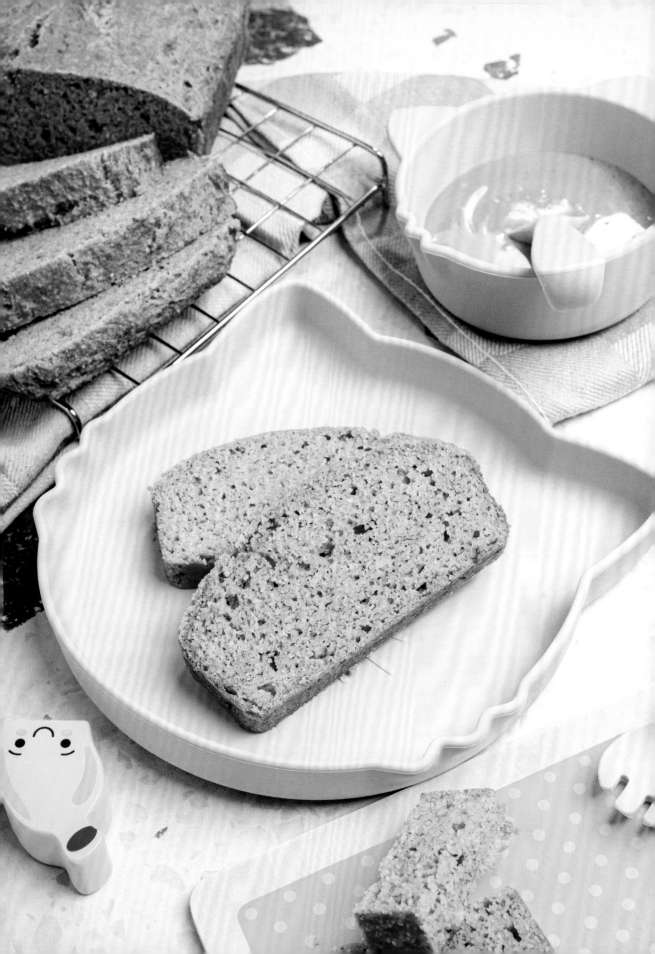

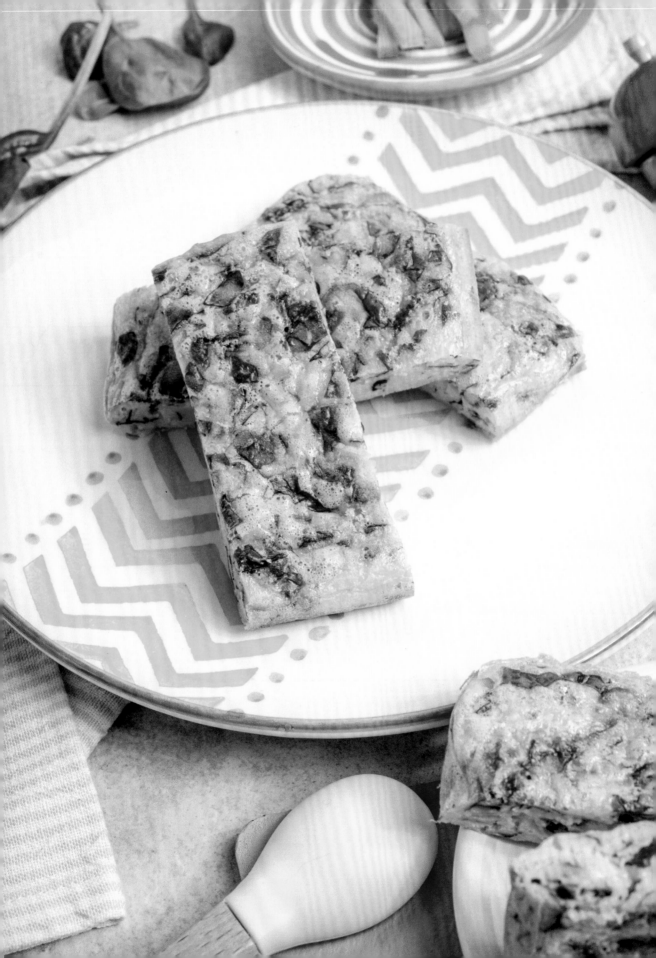

Spinach Egg Bake

prep **5 minutes** / cook **20 minutes** / makes **8 sticks**

⅓ cup (20 g) spinach, packed (see Tip 1)

3 large eggs

⅓ cup (43 g) all-purpose flour

⅓ cup (38 g) shredded cheddar (see Tip 2)

½ teaspoon baking powder

¼ teaspoon onion powder

¼ teaspoon salt (optional)

This protein-packed egg bake is an effortless way to get a serving of eggs and veggies in the morning. It's simple to prepare and can be customized with your favorite veggies and other mix-ins for different flavor combinations. Slicing it into strips makes it easier for little ones to manage and eat.

1 Preheat the oven to 350°F (180°C). Line a 9 × 5-inch (23 × 13 cm) loaf pan with parchment paper.

2 Finely chop the spinach leaves and set aside.

3 Whisk the eggs in a large bowl until the yolks and whites are fully incorporated.

4 Add the flour, cheddar, baking powder, onion powder, and salt (if using), and whisk into a thick mixture.

5 Stir in the chopped spinach leaves, and pour the mixture into the loaf pan.

6 Bake for 20 minutes, or until the edges are lightly golden and the top is firm.

7 Let cool completely in the pan, slice into eight sticks, and serve.

Storage

Store cooled sticks in an airtight container in the fridge for up to 4 days. To freeze, store in a freezer-safe bag with most of the air removed for up to 3 months. To reheat, microwave for 20 seconds, adding 10-second increments as needed, until warmed through.

Tips

1. Replace the spinach with different veggies or fillings, such as finely chopped broccoli, bell peppers, onions, and bacon, for some fun flavor variations!

2. Shredded cheddar cheese provides a great, bold flavor in this egg bake. If preparing this for a young baby, mozzarella is a nice low-sodium alternative.

Blackberry Cheesecake French Toast Sticks

prep **8 minutes** / cook **5 minutes** / makes **6 to 8 sticks**

4 slices sandwich bread

¼ cup (37 g) blackberries

2 tablespoons cream cheese, softened (see Tip 1)

1 egg (see Tip 2)

3 tablespoons milk

¼ teaspoon ground cinnamon

¼ teaspoon vanilla extract

1 to 2 tablespoons unsalted butter

Maple syrup, for serving (optional, see Tip 3)

French toast is already a decadent treat, but stuffed French toast takes this breakfast classic to the next level! These French toast sticks are oozing with blackberry and cream cheese goodness. They are a naturally sweetened breakfast treat and only take a few minutes to prepare. These will soon become a go-to meal that the whole family will love.

1 Cut the crusts off the slices of bread.

2 Mash the blackberries in a small bowl and set aside.

3 Spread the cream cheese on two slices of bread (1 tablespoon per slice), then top each slice with an equal amount of mashed blackberries.

4 Place the remaining slices of bread on top of the blackberries to form two sandwiches. Slice the sandwiches into three or four sticks.

5 Whisk together the egg, milk, cinnamon, and vanilla extract in a large bowl until well combined.

6 Melt the butter in a medium frying pan over medium-low heat.

7 Dip the French toast sticks into the batter, shaking off any excess, and cook until golden brown on all edges, a few minutes per side.

8 Serve with a side of maple syrup, if using.

Storage

Store in an airtight container in the fridge for up to 2 days. To freeze, store in a freezer-safe bag with most of the air removed for up to 3 months. To reheat, microwave for 20 to 30 seconds, until warmed through. You can also reheat them in a toaster until warmed through.

Tips

1. Feel free to swap the cream cheese with mascarpone cheese for a lower-sodium option for your little one.

2. Egg-free? Replace the egg with a few tablespoons of unsweetened applesauce.

3. Serve to baby as is and with a drizzle of maple syrup to dip for the rest of the family!

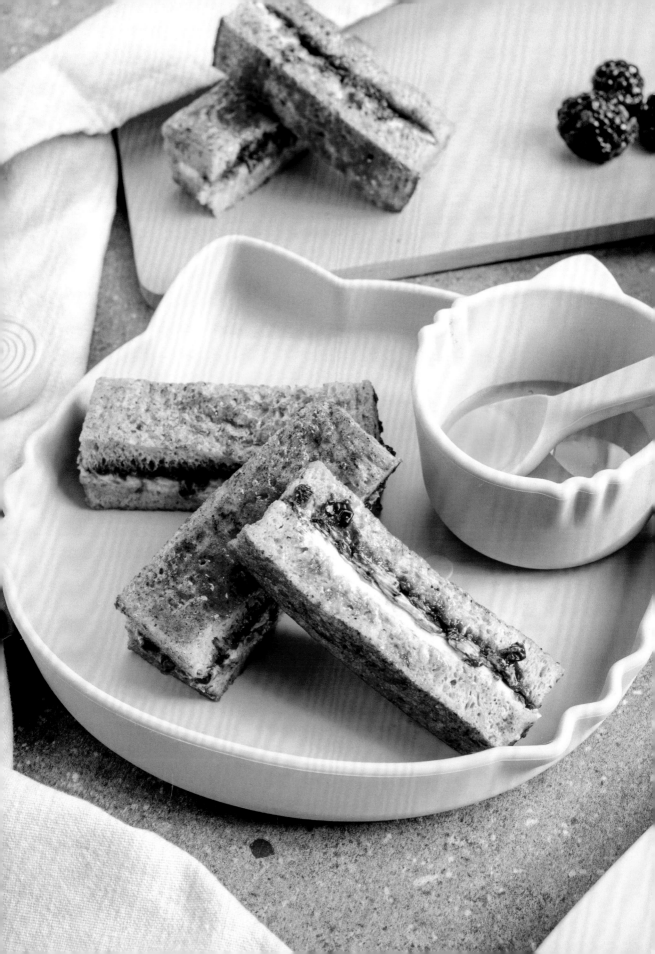

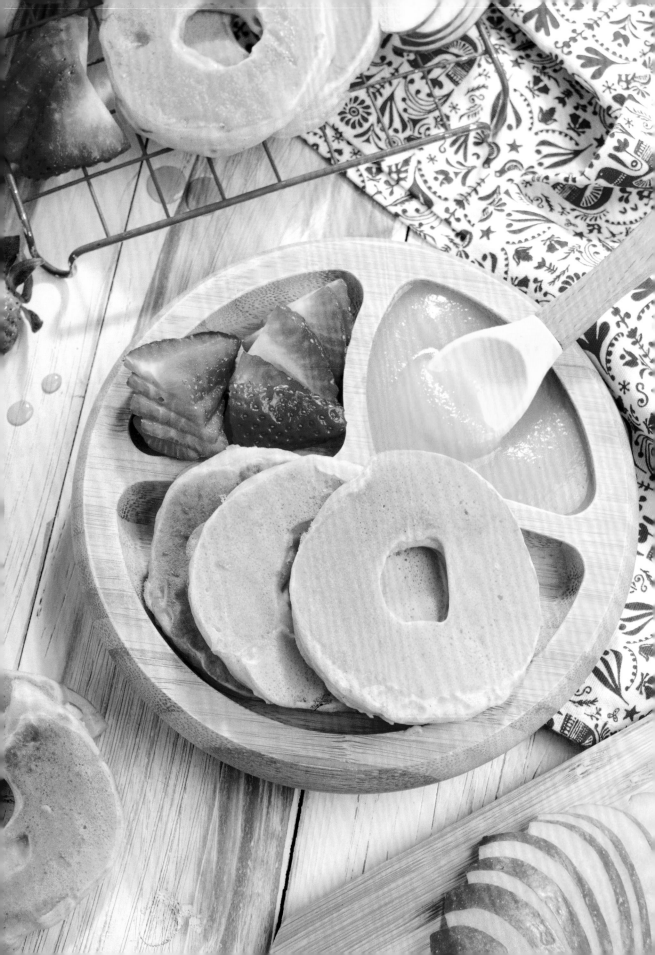

Dipped Apple Pancakes

prep **8 minutes** / cook **5 minutes** / makes **10 to 15 pancakes**

1 cup (130 g) all-purpose flour
2 teaspoons baking powder
½ teaspoon ground cinnamon
1 cup (240 ml) milk
¼ cup (60 ml) melted unsalted butter or mild-tasting oil
1 tablespoon maple syrup, plus more for serving (optional, see Tip 2)
2 large apples (preferably Honeycrisp or Fuji)
1 to 2 tablespoons unsalted butter

Pancakes are a classic, but when you fill them with apples, it's like taking a bite of apple pie for breakfast! The apples soften as they cook, and you end up with a fluffy pancake coating on top of a sweet apple slice. The apples add the perfect touch of sweetness, and the cinnamon brings warm spice to this fun breakfast treat.

1 Whisk together the flour, baking powder, and cinnamon in a large bowl until combined. Add the milk, melted butter, and maple syrup, and whisk until smooth.

2 Peel the apples, and slice them horizontally into ½-inch (1 cm) circles. Use a small measuring spoon or mini cookie cutter to remove the core from the slices.

3 Heat a medium frying pan over medium-low heat. Add the butter to the pan to melt (see Tip 1).

4 Dip the apple slices into the pancake batter, and shake off any excess. Place the dipped apples into the pan to cook.

5 When small bubbles begin to form after 2 or 3 minutes, flip the pancakes and cook until golden on the other side, 1 to 2 minutes.

6 Serve with a side of maple syrup, if using.

Storage

These dipped apple pancakes are best enjoyed fresh but can be stored in an airtight container in the fridge for up to 3 days. They can be frozen in an airtight container for up to 3 months. To reheat, microwave for 20 to 30 seconds, until warmed through.

Tips

1. If you are using a nonstick pan, you can skip the butter and cook the pancakes directly on the pan. This is the secret to perfectly browned pancakes.
2. Serve to baby as is and with a drizzle of maple syrup to dip for the rest of the family!

Overnight Oats

prep **5 minutes** / serves **1 adult & 1 child**

(EF) (GF) (NF) (V)

Pumpkin Pie Overnight Oats

1 cup (90 g) old-fashioned rolled oats

1 cup (240 ml) milk

½ cup (120 g) plain whole milk Greek yogurt

½ cup (120 g) pumpkin puree

2 tablespoons maple syrup (optional)

2 teaspoons ground chia seeds

1 teaspoon pumpkin pie spice or ground cinnamon, plus more for serving

(EF) (GF) (V)

Banana Overnight Oats

2 medium ripe bananas, mashed

1 cup (240 ml) milk

1 cup (90 g) old-fashioned rolled oats

2 tablespoons natural peanut butter

½ teaspoon ground cinnamon, plus more for serving

Toppings (optional)

Finely crushed granola

Sliced banana

Unsweetened coconut flakes

Whipped cream

Overnight oats are an easy breakfast item for busy weekday mornings. You can add all the ingredients to a container the night before, pop it in the fridge, and serve it with your favorite toppings the next morning. These recipes are so versatile; they can be customized with other fruits and add-ins for different flavor combinations. The pumpkin and banana flavors are great base recipes for thick, rich, and creamy oats.

1 Add all the ingredients for your preferred flavor of oats to an airtight container or mason jar, and stir thoroughly to combine. Place it in the fridge to soak overnight.

2 When ready to serve, give the mixture a stir to ensure that all the ingredients are incorporated. Add a splash of milk, if needed, to loosen the texture.

3 Top with a dash of cinnamon and your favorite toppings, and serve!

Storage

These overnight oats will keep fresh in an airtight container in the fridge for up to 5 days. The banana overnight oats will darken in color naturally but will still have the same taste.

Tips

1. Feel free to customize the flavor of the oats to your liking! Berries, nut butter, and ground nuts are great add-ins.

2. If you prefer warm oats, you can transfer the mixture to a saucepan over medium heat and cook, stirring, until warmed through, 2 to 3 minutes. Add an extra splash of milk as needed to loosen the mixture.

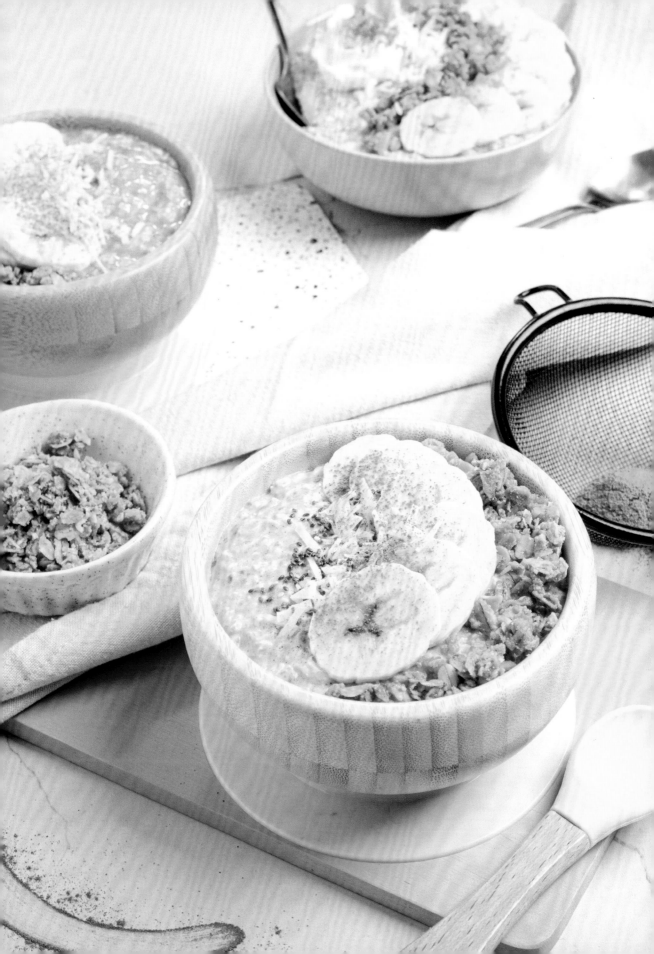

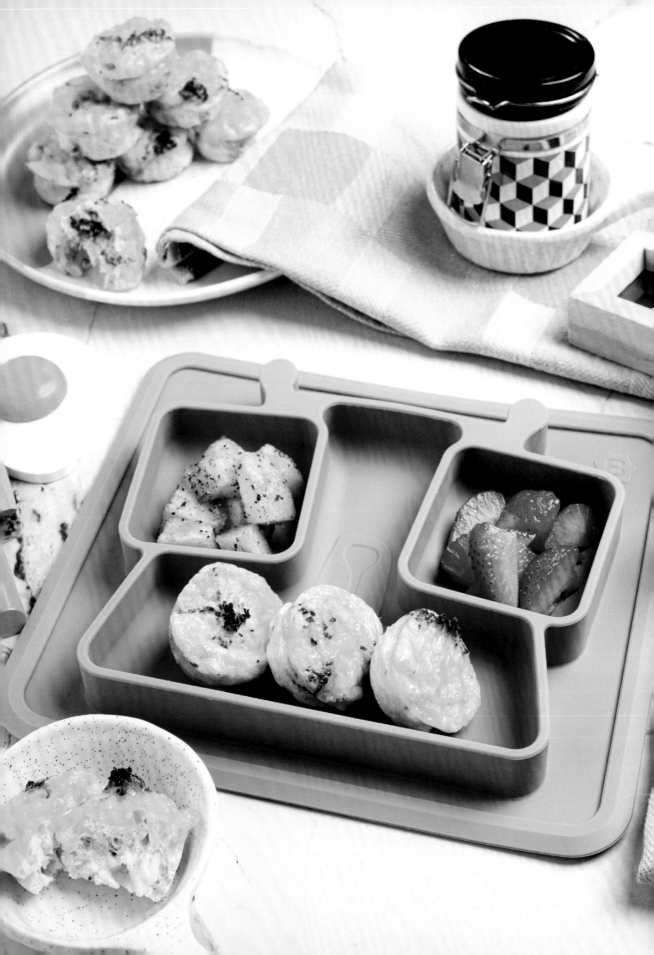

Broccoli & Cheese Egg Bites

prep **10 minutes** / cook **15 minutes** / makes **20 to 24 mini egg bites**

1 cup (90 g) broccoli
  florets
6 eggs (see Tip 1)
¾ cup (85 g) shredded
  cheddar, divided (see
  Tip 2)
¼ cup (60 ml) heavy
  cream
¼ teaspoon onion
  powder
¼ teaspoon salt (optional)
⅛ teaspoon black pepper

These egg bites are packed with broccoli and cheddar flavor—the ultimate combo! They are freezer friendly and great to meal prep, store, and reheat for a well-balanced breakfast on busy mornings. Swap the broccoli with your favorite veggies for an iron- and vitamin C–packed morning fix.

1 Preheat the oven to 350°F (180°C).

2 Place the broccoli florets in a microwave-safe bowl with 1 tablespoon of water and microwave for 3 minutes, or until fork-tender. (You can also steam the broccoli in a steamer basket for 10 minutes, or until tender.) Drain the liquid, and use kitchen scissors or a knife to finely chop the broccoli.

3 Whisk the eggs in a medium bowl. Add ½ cup (57 g) cheddar, heavy cream, onion powder, salt (if using), and pepper, and whisk until combined.

4 Add about 1 teaspoon of chopped broccoli into each cup of a 24-cup mini-muffin pan (see Tip 3).

5 Pour about 1 tablespoon of the egg mixture into each mini-muffin cup. Evenly distribute the remaining cheddar over the top of the egg mixture.

6 Bake the bites for about 15 minutes, or until a toothpick inserted into the center comes out clean.

7 Let cool completely in the pan, and serve.

Storage

Store in an airtight container in the fridge for up to 4 days. To freeze, store in a freezer-safe bag with most of the air removed for up to 3 months. To reheat, microwave the bites for 15 to 20 seconds, until warmed through.

Tips

1. Egg-free? Replace the eggs with a liquid egg substitute like JUST Egg.
2. Dairy-free? Swap the cheese and heavy cream with dairy-free cheese shreds and a dairy-free milk alternative.
3. Use a silicone mini-muffin pan so that the egg bites pop right out! If you use a silicone pan, place it on top of a baking sheet for easy transferring into and out of the oven. If you use a normal pan, be sure to spray the cups with cooking spray before adding the broccoli and egg mixture.

Banana French Toast

prep **5 minutes** / cook **5 minutes** / serves **1 adult & 1 child**

1 small overripe banana

1 egg (see Tip 1)

¼ teaspoon ground cinnamon

¼ teaspoon vanilla extract

1 tablespoon coconut oil

3 to 4 slices sourdough bread

Maple syrup, for serving (optional, see Tip 2)

This French toast recipe is made with minimal ingredients and sweetened with overripe bananas. I love using sourdough bread for this because it really absorbs the custard liquids for a bite that's crisp on the outside and soft on the inside.

1 Mash the banana in a large bowl until smooth.

2 Add the egg, cinnamon, and vanilla extract, and whisk until well combined.

3 Heat a medium frying pan over medium-low heat, and add the oil.

4 Dip the bread slices into the batter, and shake off any excess. Add the slices to the pan in batches, and cook until golden on both sides, 2 to 3 minutes per side.

5 Serve with a side of maple syrup, if using.

Storage

Store in an airtight container in the fridge for up to 2 days. To freeze, store in a freezer-safe bag with most of the air removed for up to 1 month. To reheat, microwave for 20 to 30 seconds, until warmed through.

Tips

1. Egg-free? Replace the egg with 2 tablespoons of milk or unsweetened applesauce.

2. Serve to baby as is and with a drizzle of maple syrup for the rest of the family!

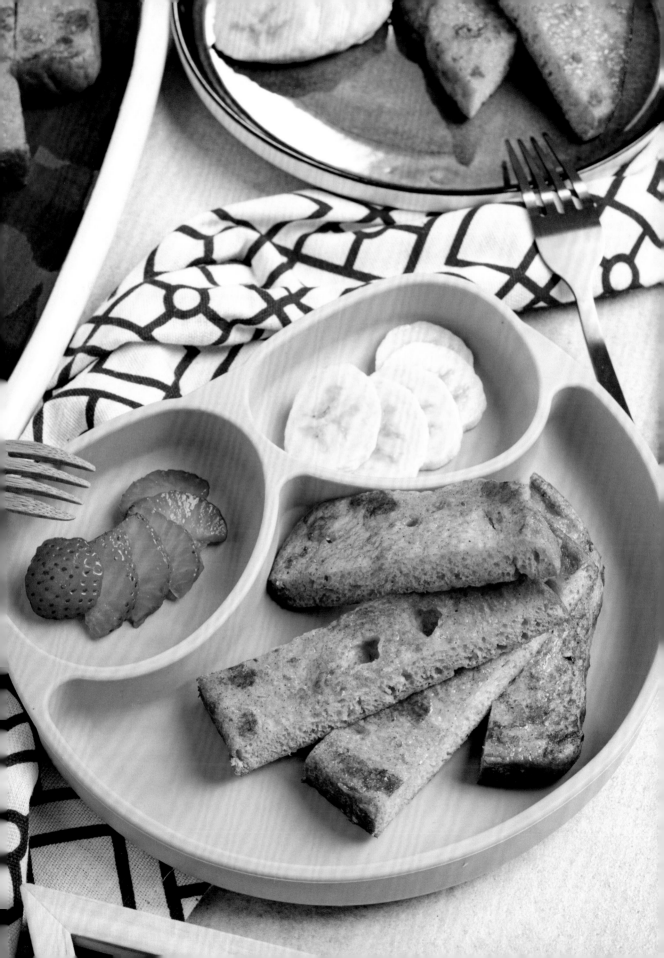

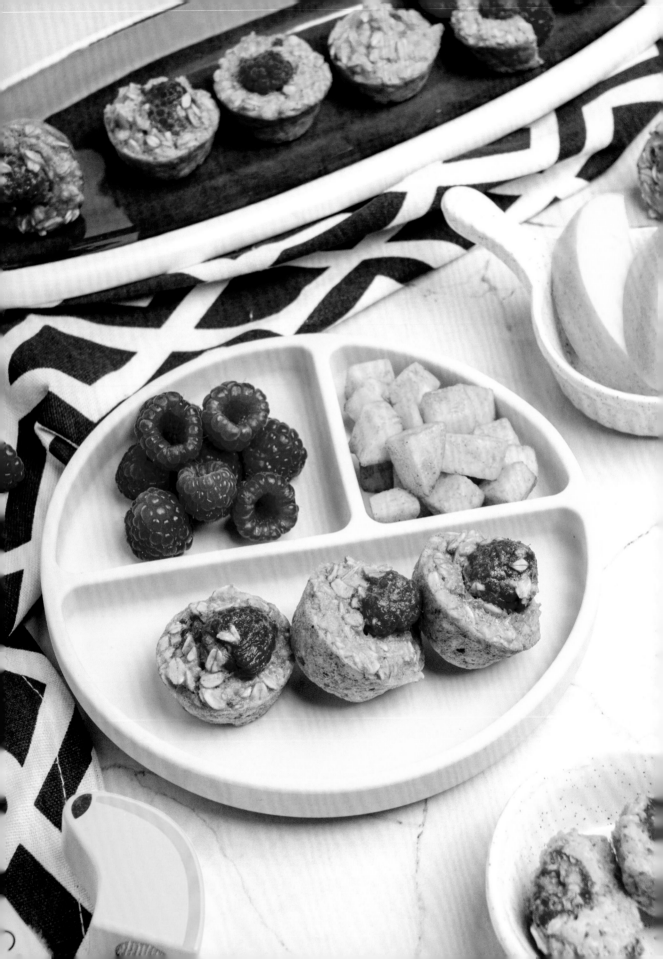

Raspberry Oat Bites

prep **10 minutes** / cook **15 minutes** / makes **16 to 20 mini oat bites**

1 large overripe banana

⅓ cup (80 ml) milk
(see Tip 1)

1 egg (see Tip 2)

¼ teaspoon ground
cinnamon

¼ teaspoon vanilla
extract

1 cup (90 g) old-fashioned
rolled oats

½ cup (75 g) raspberries

These little bites are one of my favorite things to bake on the weekends, refrigerate or freeze, and reheat for breakfast throughout the week. I make them with all different types of fruits so my boys have variety in flavor while still getting a great serving of fiber and nutrients. Raspberries add the perfect tartness to balance out the natural sweetness of the banana.

1 Preheat the oven to 350°F (180°C).

2 Blend the banana, milk, egg, cinnamon, and vanilla extract in a blender until smooth. Pour the mixture into a medium bowl.

3 Add the oats, and stir until combined. Stir in the raspberries.

4 Spoon tablespoon-sized portions of batter into a 24-cup silicone mini-muffin pan (see Tip 3).

5 Bake for 15 to 18 minutes, until cooked through.

6 Let the oat bites cool completely to firm up before removing them from the pan.

Storage

Store in an airtight container at room temperature for up to 2 days or in the fridge for up to 5 days. To freeze, store in a freezer-safe bag with most of the air removed for up to 3 months. To reheat, microwave for 20 to 30 seconds, until warmed through.

Tips

1. Dairy-free? Replace the milk with a dairy-free alternative like coconut milk or oat milk.

2. Egg-free? Swap the egg with a flax egg (see page 55).

3. Do not use paper liners for these oat bites because they will stick. If using a metal mini-muffin pan, grease the pan with cooking spray so the bites won't stick.

Fluffy Cheesy Scrambled Eggs

prep **3 minutes** / cook **5 minutes** / serves **1 adult & 1 child**

4 large eggs
¼ cup (60 ml) half-and-half
¼ teaspoon salt (optional)
⅛ teaspoon black pepper
1 tablespoon unsalted butter
¼ cup (28 g) shredded cheddar

If you've been looking for a great scrambled egg recipe, look no further! These eggs are soft and fluffy, and the added cheese makes them so much more satisfying. The cheddar has a nice, bold flavor, but the special ingredient here is half-and-half, which adds so much creaminess. When cooked low and slow, these cheesy eggs come out perfect every time.

1 Add the eggs, half-and-half, salt (if using), and pepper to a large bowl, and whisk until smooth with the yolk and whites fully incorporated.

2 Melt the butter in a small pan over medium-low heat.

3 Add the egg mixture to the pan. As the edges begin to firm up and set after a few seconds, use a spatula to push in the edges, tilting the pan around so the liquid in the center can pool to the edges and set.

4 Cook until the eggs are mostly cooked, 3 to 5 minutes, and then gently fold the eggs onto each other and bring them together in the center of the pan.

5 Turn off the heat, sprinkle the cheddar over the eggs, and gently fold again so the cheddar melts and incorporates into the eggs. (The retained heat in the pan will melt the cheese.)

6 Let cool completely before serving.

Storage

These scrambled eggs are best enjoyed fresh but can be stored in an airtight container in the fridge for up to 3 days. If storing, be sure to refrigerate within 2 hours.

Note

· This is a great base recipe for scrambled eggs. Feel free to add some variety by mixing in some add-ins. Chopped bell peppers, onions, spinach, and bacon are great options to add some flavor and texture.

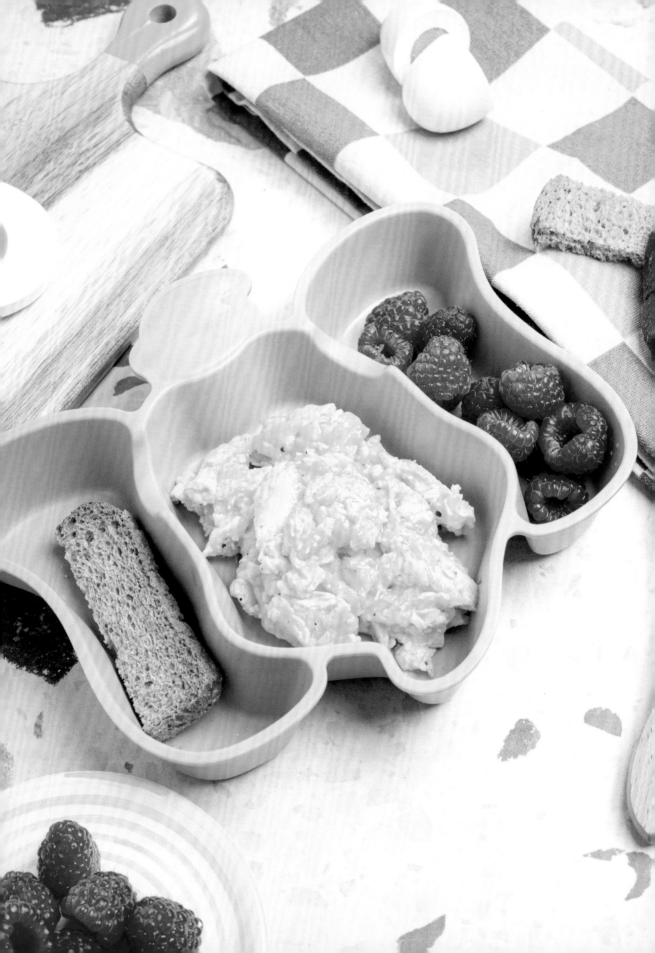

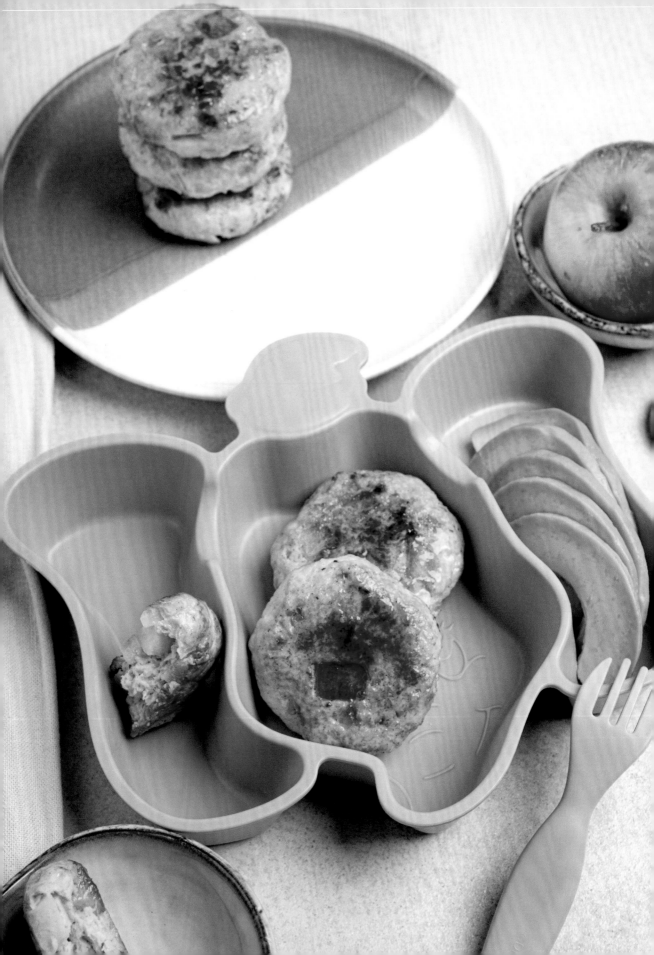

Chicken & Apple Breakfast Sausage

prep **8 minutes** / cook **8 minutes** / makes **9 patties**

1 pound (454 g) ground chicken

1 large apple, finely chopped (preferably Honeycrisp; see Tip)

½ medium yellow onion, finely chopped

1 tablespoon maple syrup (optional, for a sweeter sausage)

1 teaspoon garlic powder

½ teaspoon ground cinnamon

1 teaspoon salt (optional)

1 tablespoon mild-tasting oil

Chicken and apples may sound like a strange pairing, but something about the sweet and savory combination works so well. This sausage is made with simple, fresh ingredients and is moist, juicy, and subtly sweet from the apples. It's the perfect protein to serve with eggs or potatoes for breakfast. And because it's free of all the top allergens, it's a great allergy-friendly protein option.

1 Add the chicken, apple, onion, maple syrup (if using), garlic powder, cinnamon, and salt (if using) to a large bowl. Use your hands to mix the ingredients until well combined.

2 Wet your hands, then scoop out 2 tablespoon-sized portions. Form the portions into small patties, making sure that your hands remain moist throughout the process so the mixture does not stick.

3 Heat the oil in a large nonstick pan over medium-low heat.

4 Add the patties to the pan in batches, and cook until golden brown, 3 to 4 minutes per side. Check on the patties at the 3-minute mark to ensure that the heat is not too high.

5 Let cool completely before serving.

Storage

Store in an airtight container in the fridge for up to 5 days. To freeze, store in a freezer-safe container for up to 2 months. To reheat, microwave for 15 to 20 seconds, until warmed through. You can also add 1 tablespoon of water to a hot frying pan over medium-low heat and reheat the frozen patties, covered, for 2 to 3 minutes total.

Tip

· If preparing these for a baby, be sure to finely chop the apples so they fully soften as they cook and there are no large chunks for baby to potentially choke on.

Strawberry Oatmeal Bars

prep **10 minutes** / cook **25 minutes** / makes **8 bars**

¼ cup (60 g) plain whole milk Greek yogurt

3 tablespoons unsalted butter, melted

2 tablespoons maple syrup

⅔ cup (60 g) old-fashioned rolled oats

⅔ cup (67 g) almond flour (see Tip 1)

¼ teaspoon ground cinnamon

½ cup (75 g) chopped strawberries

When I have some strawberries on hand that are about to go bad, I love turning them into several batches of these bars. My boys are obsessed with strawberries, but occasionally I overestimate how much they'll eat and end up with a stash that needs to be consumed quickly. These bars are made with hearty oats as the base and have bursts of sweet strawberry. They are a great way to get in a serving of fruit and oats in the morning in a filling breakfast treat!

1 Preheat the oven to 350°F (180°C). Line a 9 × 5-inch (23 × 13 cm) loaf pan with parchment paper (see Tip 2).

2 Whisk the yogurt, butter, and maple syrup in a large bowl to form a smooth custard with no lumps.

3 Add the oats, almond flour, and cinnamon, and stir until combined into a thick mixture. Fold in the strawberries.

4 Transfer the mixture to the loaf pan, and use a spatula to smooth it into a flat, even layer.

5 Bake for 25 minutes, or until the edges are slightly golden brown and the top is firm and set.

6 Let cool completely in the pan before removing and slicing into eight squares.

Storage

Store in an airtight container at room temperature for up to 3 days. To freeze, store in a freezer-safe container for up to 3 months. To reheat, microwave for 20 to 30 seconds, until warmed through.

Tips

1. Nut-free? Replace the almond flour with oat flour. The bars will be denser in texture and will not be as moist, but they'll have a similar taste.

2. This recipe doubles well. Bake in a 9-inch (23 cm) square pan for the same amount of time.

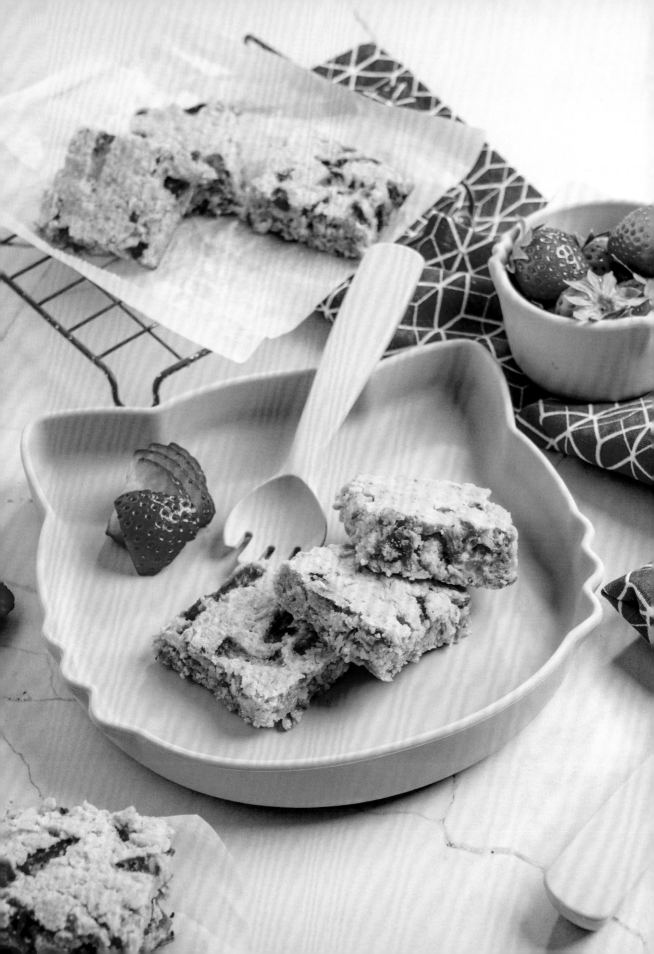

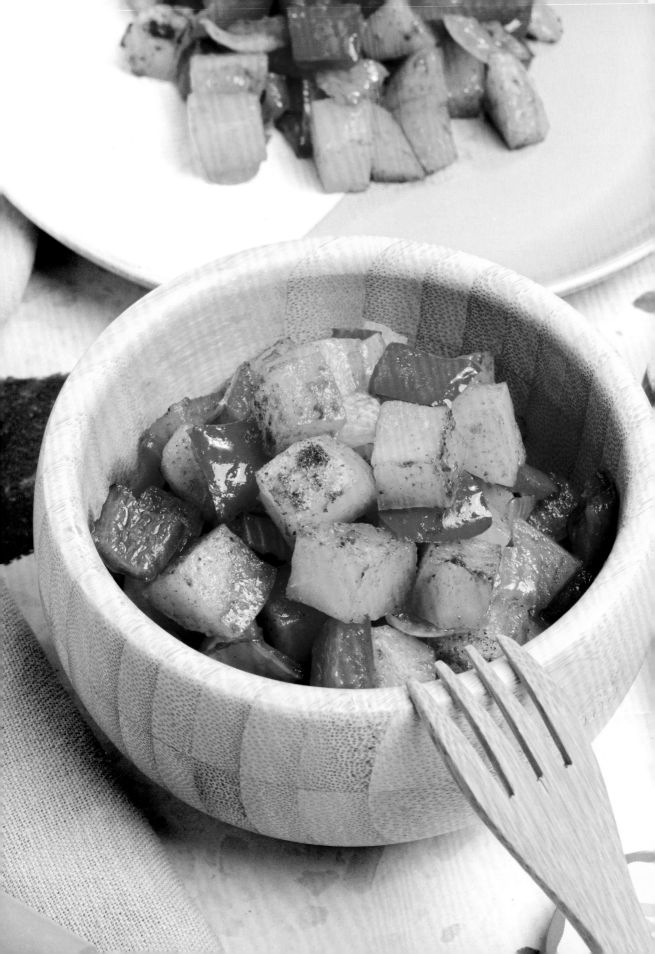

Oven-Roasted Breakfast Potatoes

prep **10 minutes** / cook **35 minutes** / serves **2 adults & 2 children**

2 pounds (907 g) Yukon Gold potatoes

½ small red bell pepper, ribs and seeds removed

½ small green bell pepper, ribs and seeds removed

1 small yellow onion

1 teaspoon sweet paprika

½ teaspoon garlic powder

1 teaspoon salt (optional, see Tip 1)

2 tablespoons olive oil

These breakfast potatoes are the perfect side to go with your favorite morning protein. Yukon Gold potatoes yield perfectly velvety and buttery potatoes, and bell peppers and onions add extra texture and flavor. Prep everything in one dish, and just pop it into the oven to roast!

1 Preheat the oven to 400°F (200°C). Line a baking sheet with parchment paper.

2 Peel the potatoes, and dice them into ½-inch (1 cm) pieces (see Tip 2).

3 Rinse the potatoes with cold water, drain, and pat dry. Place them in a large bowl.

4 Dice the bell peppers and onion into ½-inch (1 cm) cubes, and add them to the bowl.

5 Add the paprika, garlic powder, salt (if using), and oil, and toss to coat the vegetables evenly.

6 Transfer the mixture to the baking sheet, spread into a single layer, and bake for 35 minutes, stirring after 20 minutes, until the potatoes are golden and slightly crisp and the onions and peppers are tender.

7 Let cool before serving.

Storage

These potatoes are best enjoyed fresh but can be stored in an airtight container in the fridge for up to 2 days. To reheat, bake at 350°F (180°C) for 10 to 15 minutes, until warmed through.

Tips

1. Before adding salt, remove baby's portion, then sprinkle some salt on the remaining potato mixture for the rest of the family. You can cook baby's portion on the same baking sheet in a separate corner of the pan.

2. If your little one has not yet mastered the pincer grasp, cut a few potatoes into finger-sized strips to make them easier to pick up and hold.

Blueberry Sheet Pan Pancakes

prep **10 minutes** / cook **18 minutes** / makes **24 slices**

2 cups (260 g) all-purpose flour (see Tip 1)

2 teaspoons baking powder

1 teaspoon ground cinnamon

2 eggs (see Tip 2)

1 cup (240 ml) milk

4 tablespoons unsalted butter, melted and cooled

¼ cup (60 ml) maple syrup (optional; see Tip 3)

1 teaspoon vanilla extract

1 cup (150 g) blueberries, plus more to sprinkle on top (see Tip 4)

I know I can't be the only one who loves the idea of being able to feed a crowd without having to stand at the stove forever. These sheet pan pancakes are the perfect way to batch-make pancakes without having to worry about the constant flipping. They're simple to make and easily customizable with your favorite toppings and add-ins.

1 Preheat the oven to 400°F (200°C). Line a 10 × 15-inch (27 × 39 cm) baking sheet with parchment paper.

2 Whisk together the flour, baking powder, and cinnamon in a large bowl.

3 Whisk together the eggs, milk, butter, maple syrup (if using), and vanilla extract in a medium bowl until smooth.

4 Add the wet ingredients to the bowl with the dry ingredients, and mix until just combined. Stir in the blueberries.

5 Pour the batter onto the baking sheet, and smooth it into an even layer to fill the entire pan. Sprinkle a few more blueberries on top.

6 Bake for 16 to 18 minutes, until a knife inserted into the center comes out clean.

7 Let cool completely before slicing into 24 rectangles.

Storage

Store in an airtight container in the fridge for up to 2 days. To freeze, store in a freezer-safe bag with most of the air removed for up to 1 month. To reheat, microwave for 20 to 30 seconds, until warmed through. You can also place on a baking sheet and reheat in a 350°F (180°C) oven for 5 to 10 minutes, until warmed through.

Tips

1. Gluten-free? Swap the all-purpose flour with a gluten-free flour blend.

2. Egg-free? Replace the eggs with an extra 1 cup (240 ml) of milk combined with 2 tablespoons of lemon juice and add 2 more teaspoons of baking powder with the dry ingredients. Bake this egg-free version at 425°F (220°C) for 16 to 18 minutes.

3. If preparing these for a baby, omit the maple syrup from the batter and serve it on the side for everyone else.

4. Swap the blueberries with your favorite fruits, add-ins, or toppings. When serving fresh blueberries to babies or young toddlers, quarter or smash them into discs to eliminate roundness. Whole, uncooked blueberries are a choking hazard.

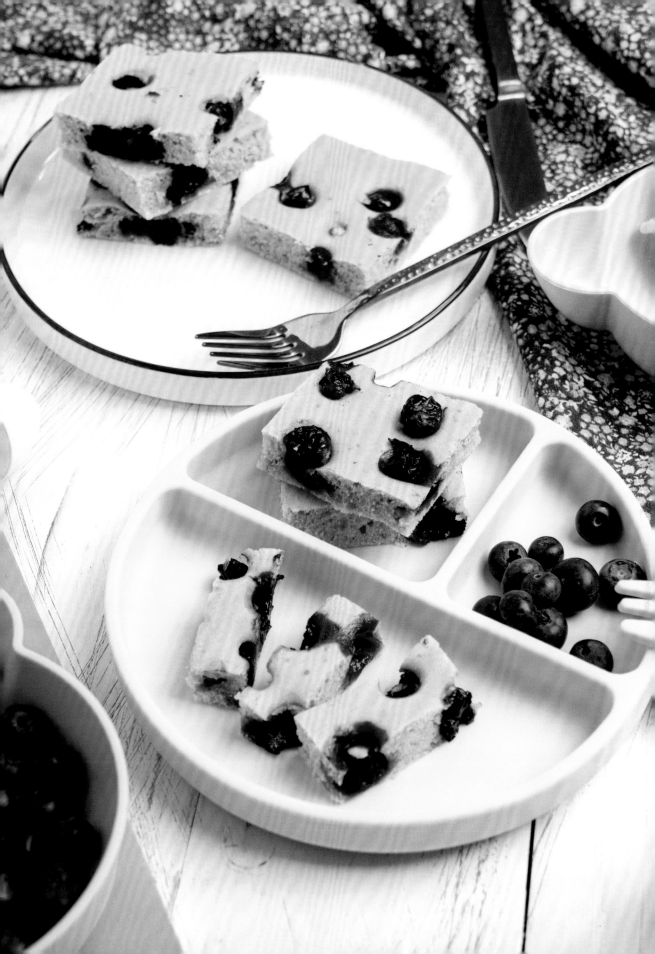

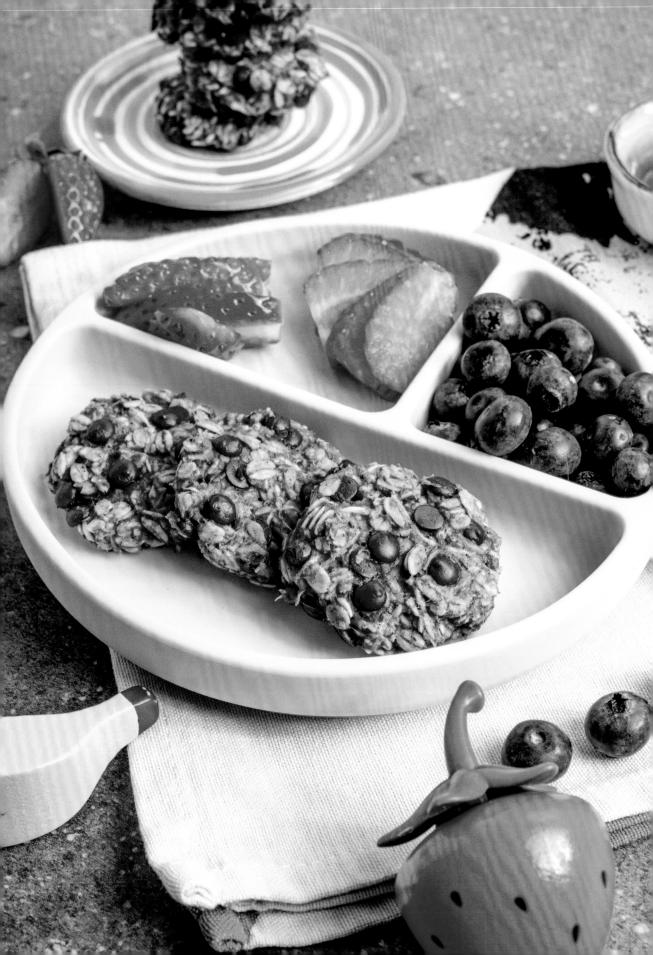

Zucchini Banana Cookies

prep **8 minutes** / cook **10 minutes** / makes **14 cookies**

½ cup (110 g) packed finely grated zucchini

1 large overripe banana

2 tablespoons natural peanut butter

¾ cup (68 g) old-fashioned rolled oats

½ teaspoon ground cinnamon

¼ cup (43 g) mini chocolate chips (optional, see Tip)

Did someone say cookies for breakfast? Yes, please! These cookies are a soft and sweet, filling treat—and a great way to get in a serving of veggies. They are made with rolled oats, which will keep your little one feeling full. They're naturally sweetened with bananas, and you can fold in some chocolate chips for an extra treat!

1 Preheat the oven to 350°F (180°C). Line a baking sheet with parchment paper.

2 Use a cheesecloth, a clean kitchen towel, or your hands to squeeze out as much moisture from the zucchini as possible. You should end up with about ¼ cup (45 g) of zucchini.

3 Mash the banana in a large bowl until smooth. Add the peanut butter, and mix until smooth.

4 Add the oats, zucchini, and cinnamon to the bowl, and mix until well combined. Fold in the chocolate chips, if using.

5 Scoop out heaping tablespoon-sized portions of the batter and place on the baking sheet. Flatten the portions, and shape into cookies. (They will not change shape while baking, so be sure to flatten them to your preferred thickness.)

6 Bake for 10 minutes, or until the cookies are firm and set.

7 Let cool completely before serving.

Storage

Store in an airtight container at room temperature for up to 2 days or in the refrigerator for up to 5 days. To freeze, store in a freezer-safe bag with most of the air removed for up to 2 months. To reheat, microwave for 10 to 15 seconds, until warmed through. You can also thaw completely at room temperature for 1 to 2 hours.

Tip

- Form cookies with half of the batter for baby, and add the mini chocolate chips to the rest of the mixture for everyone else!

Mixed Berry French Toast Bake

prep **10 minutes** / cook **35 minutes** / makes **6 slices**

Cooking spray (olive or avocado oil)

5 to 6 slices of bread (see Tip 1)

¾ cup (113 g) mixed berries, divided

1 large overripe banana

2 eggs (see Tip 2)

⅓ cup (80 ml) milk

½ teaspoon ground cinnamon

½ teaspoon vanilla extract

This French toast bake is sweetened with just blueberries and bananas. It is the perfect make-ahead breakfast treat that the whole family can enjoy! The French toast is moist and perfect for baby-led weaning.

1 Preheat the oven to 350°F (180°C). Grease a 9 × 5-inch (23 × 13 cm) loaf pan with cooking spray.

2 Cut the bread slices into 1-inch (2.5 cm) squares (you should have about 4 cups/160 g), and add half of them to the pan.

3 Finely dice the berries, and sprinkle ½ cup (75 g) into the pan with the bread. Top with the remaining bread squares.

4 Blend together the banana, eggs, milk, cinnamon, and vanilla extract in a blender to form the batter.

5 Pour the batter on top of the bread and berries in the pan. Press down gently on the bread pieces to submerge into the batter, and top with the remaining chopped berries (see Tip 3).

6 Bake for 35 minutes, or until golden and dry to the touch.

7 Let cool completely before serving.

Storage

Store in an airtight container in the fridge for up to 2 days. I like to section out and wrap individual portions to reheat easily when ready to serve. To freeze, store the individually wrapped portions in a freezer-safe bag with most of the air removed for up to 2 months. To reheat, place on a baking sheet and bake in a 350°F (180°C) oven for 8 to 10 minutes, until warmed through. You can also microwave for a few seconds, until warmed through.

Tips

1. Slightly stale, dry, or firm bread works best for this recipe because it both holds its shape when cut (see step 2) and soaks up the batter better.

2. Egg-free? Swap the eggs with ¼ cup (63 g) of unsweetened applesauce and an extra ¼ cup (60 ml) of milk.

3. If time permits, prep this bake the night before, cover it with plastic wrap, and place it in the fridge overnight so the bread can soak up all the batter. Bake the next morning as directed.

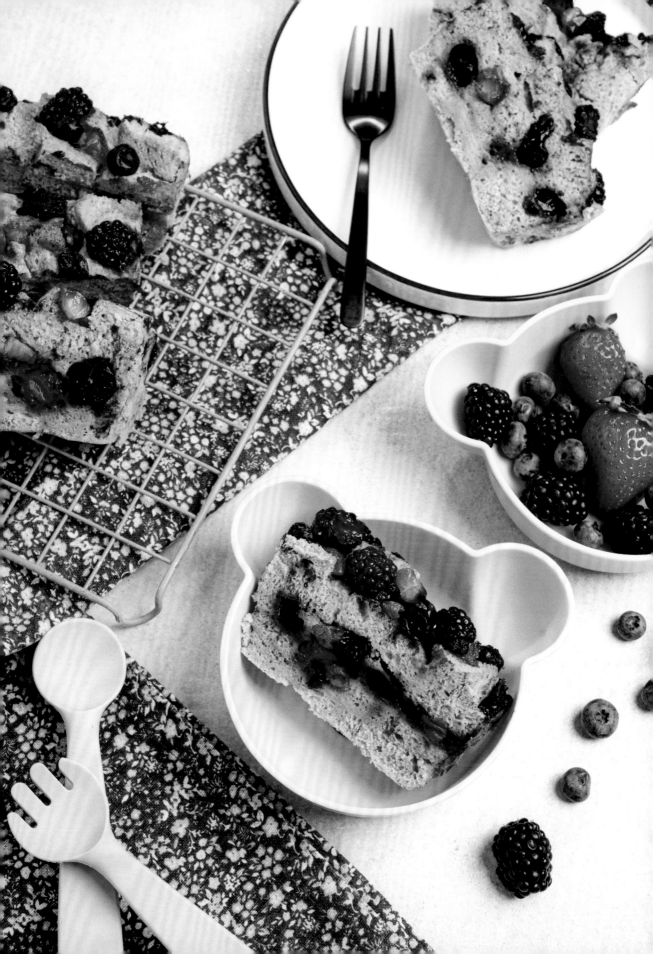

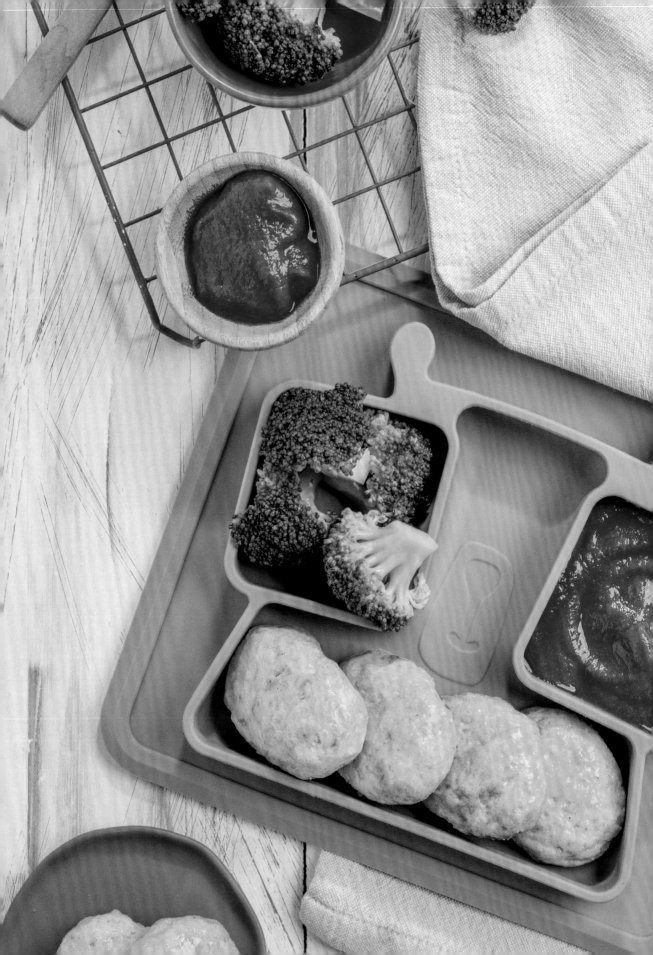

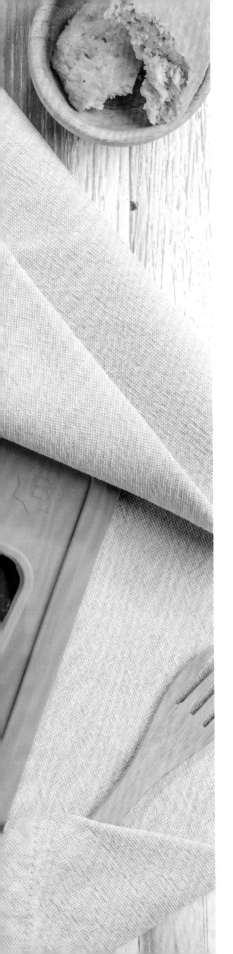

Lunch

It's lunchtime; you've made it through the hectic morning and need a quick midday meal to offer your little one. Or maybe your child is in school and you're looking for options to make ahead and pack in their lunch box. This chapter is filled with lunch options that take only a few minutes to prepare and store well to serve on another day. From easy-to-make finger foods to simple sandwiches and flatbreads, I've got you covered with these lunch ideas that the whole family will enjoy!

Cheddar Broccoli Fritters

prep **8 minutes** / cook **5 minutes** / makes **16 mini fritters**

3 cups (270 g) broccoli florets (about 2 cups chopped)

¾ cup (85 g) mild-tasting shredded cheddar

1 egg (see Tip 1)

2 tablespoons all-purpose flour

¼ teaspoon garlic powder

¼ teaspoon onion powder

¼ teaspoon salt (optional)

Mild-tasting oil, for frying

There's no denying the classic broccoli and cheese pairing. Something magical happens when you combine cheese with veggies, and that's definitely the case with these fritters. They are crisp on the outside, soft and tender on the inside, and full of cheesy goodness.

1 Place the broccoli florets in a microwave-safe bowl with 1 tablespoon of water and microwave for 3 minutes, or until fork-tender. (You can also steam the broccoli in a steamer basket for 10 minutes, or until tender.)

2 Drain the liquid, and use kitchen scissors or a knife to finely chop the broccoli (see Tip 2). Let cool completely.

3 Add the cheddar, egg, flour, garlic powder, onion powder, and salt (if using) to the bowl, and mix until well combined.

4 Heat a thin layer of oil in a large frying pan over medium heat. When the oil is hot, working in batches, scoop tablespoon-sized portions of the batter into the pan, and use the back of the spoon or a spatula to press down and flatten the fritters. Cook until golden on both sides, 2 to 3 minutes per side.

5 Transfer to a paper towel–lined plate to cool, and repeat with the remaining batter. Serve warm.

Storage

Store in an airtight container in the fridge for up to 3 days. To freeze, store in a freezer-safe bag with most of the air removed for up to 3 months. To reheat, microwave for 20 to 30 seconds, adding 10-second intervals as needed, until warmed through. You can also place on a baking sheet and reheat in a 350°F (180°C) oven for 10 minutes, or until warmed through.

Tips

1. Egg-free? Swap the egg with a flax egg (see page 55).
2. If you prefer a smoother mixture with less texture, use a food processor to chop the broccoli finely.

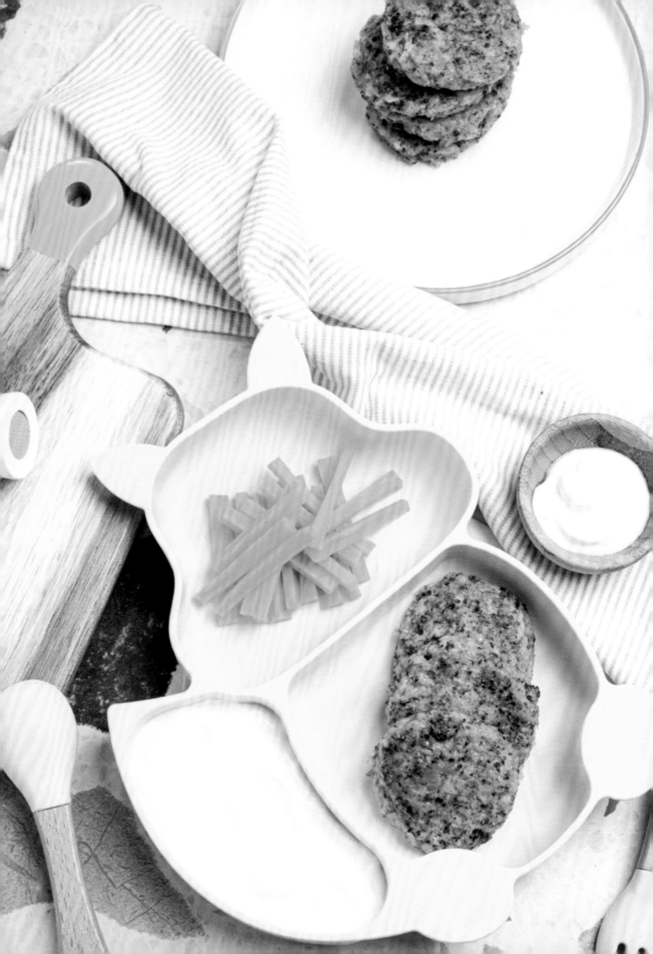

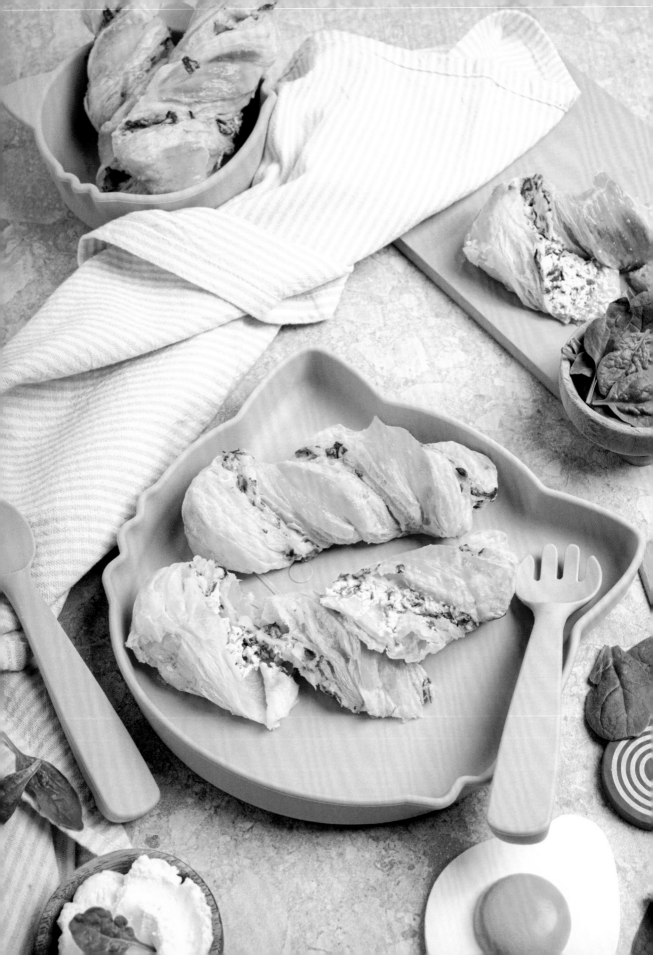

Flaky Spinach Twists

prep **8 minutes** / cook **20 minutes** / makes **8 twists**

All-purpose flour, for dusting

1 sheet puff pastry (8.6 ounces/245 g), thawed

¼ cup (15 g) baby spinach, tightly packed

¼ cup (55 g) cream cheese, softened (see Tip 1)

¼ teaspoon garlic powder

Cooking spray (olive or avocado oil, see Tip 2)

These spinach twists never last long in my house after I make them. You'll find yourself snacking on one, then two, and before you know it, the whole batch disappears. The flakiness of puff pastry combined with a creamy, cheesy filling makes for the perfect combo. They're a great way to incorporate spinach into a filling lunch!

1 Preheat the oven to 400°F (200°C). Line a baking sheet with parchment paper.

2 Dust a work surface with flour and then unfold the puff pastry sheet onto the surface so that the longer edge is on the bottom.

3 Finely chop the spinach and set aside.

4 Mix the cream cheese and garlic powder in a medium bowl until well combined. Add the spinach, and mix until incorporated.

5 Spread the spinach mixture evenly onto the bottom half of the puff pastry. Fold the top half of the pastry over the filled bottom half, and press down on the edges to seal them closed.

6 Use a pizza slicer or a knife to slice the pastry vertically into eight equal rectangular strips about 1 inch (2.5 cm) wide. Twist the ends of each strip in opposite directions twice.

7 Spray each twist generously with oil, and place them on the baking sheet.

8 Bake for 18 to 20 minutes, until golden. Serve warm.

Storage

Store in an airtight container in the fridge for up to 3 days. To freeze, store in a freezer-safe bag with most of the air removed for up to 1 month. To reheat, place on a baking sheet and bake in a 350°F (180°C) oven for 10 minutes, or until warmed through.

Tips

1. If your cream cheese is cold and you're in a hurry, you can microwave it for 10 to 15 seconds to quickly soften it. Feel free to swap cream cheese with mascarpone cheese for a lower-sodium option.
2. For a shinier crust, use an egg wash in place of the cooking spray. To make an egg wash, whisk together one egg with 1 tablespoon of water until combined and brush it onto the twists.

Cheesy Cauliflower Flatbread

prep **8 minutes** / cook **25 minutes** / makes **8 to 10 slices**

One 12-ounce (340 g) package riced cauliflower (about 2½ cups)

1¼ cups (140 g) shredded mozzarella, divided

¼ cup (25 g) grated Parmesan

1 large egg (see Tip 1)

¼ teaspoon garlic powder

¼ teaspoon Italian seasoning

¼ teaspoon salt (optional)

Marinara sauce, for serving

Cauliflower is often underrated when compared to broccoli, but it is just as nutritious! Cauliflower can be a little bland on its own, but when flavored well, it makes the most delicious dishes. Riced cauliflower is used as the base for this cheesy flatbread, and I promise that this will become your new favorite flatbread recipe. Everything comes together in one bowl and can be customized with your preferred toppings.

1 Preheat the oven to 425°F (220°C). Line a 9 × 13-inch (23 × 33 cm) baking pan with parchment paper.

2 Steam the cauliflower rice in the microwave for 2 to 3 minutes if fresh, or according to the package directions if frozen. Drain any liquid, transfer the cauliflower to a large bowl, and let cool completely.

3 Add ¾ cup (85 g) mozzarella, Parmesan, egg, garlic powder, Italian seasoning, and salt (if using) to the bowl, and mix to combine.

4 Transfer the mixture to the baking pan, and use a spatula to smooth it into a flat, even layer, pressing down well to ensure that the mixture is packed smoothly with no holes.

5 Bake for 20 minutes, or until dry to the touch.

6 Sprinkle the remaining mozzarella evenly over the top, return to the oven, and bake for 5 more minutes, or until the cheese fully melts.

7 For golden brown cheese, broil for 1 minute, keeping a close eye on it to ensure it doesn't burn.

8 Let cool, and cut into eight to ten slices (see Tip 2). Serve with marinara sauce for dipping.

Storage

Store in an airtight container in the fridge for up to 2 days. To freeze, store in a freezer-safe container for up to 1 month. To reheat, microwave for 20 to 30 seconds, adding 10-second increments as needed, until warmed through. You can also place on a baking sheet and reheat in a 350°F (180°C) oven for 10 minutes, or until warmed through.

Tips

1. Egg-free? Replace the egg with a flax egg (see page 55).
2. Slice the flatbread into thin strips to make it easier for a baby to hold.

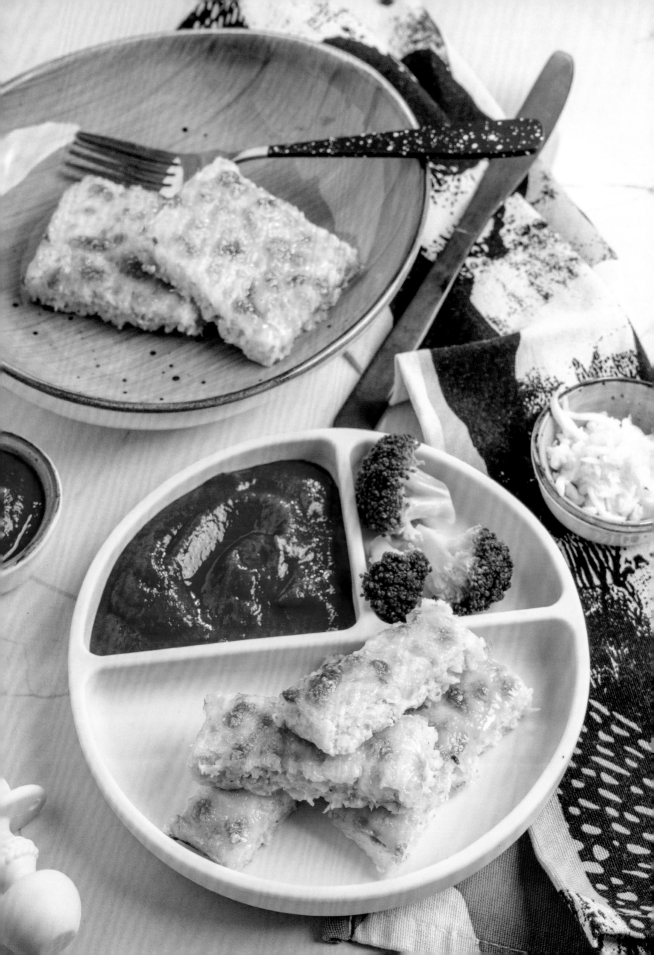

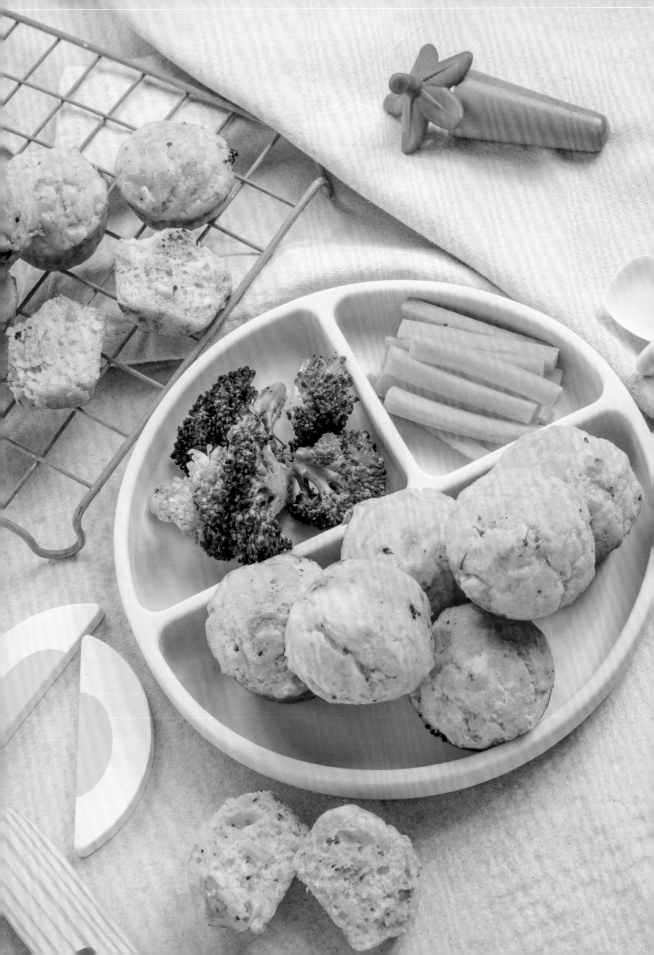

Savory Vegetable Muffins

prep **10 minutes** / cook **15 minutes** / makes **20 to 24 mini muffins**

1 egg (see Tip 1)

½ cup (120 ml) milk

¼ cup (60 ml) mild-tasting oil or melted unsalted butter

½ cup (57 g) shredded cheddar

⅓ cup (73 g) packed finely grated carrots

¼ cup (30 g) finely chopped broccoli florets

¼ cup (42 g) corn kernels

1 cup (130 g) all-purpose flour

2 teaspoons baking powder

½ teaspoon salt

⅛ teaspoon black pepper

Who says muffins have to be sweet? These vegetable muffins are savory but still as soft and fluffy as a traditional sweet muffin—like a melt-in-your-mouth biscuit. They are a great way to use up vegetables before they go bad, and you can use any veggies, cheeses, or other add-ins you have on hand. They're great warm or cold, making them a great option to pack in lunch boxes.

1 Preheat the oven to 350°F (180°C).

2 Whisk together the egg, milk, oil, and cheddar in a large bowl.

3 Add the carrots, broccoli, and corn, and mix to incorporate.

4 Add the flour, baking powder, salt, and pepper, and mix until just incorporated. It's okay if there are a few small lumps in the batter.

5 Scoop tablespoon-sized portions of batter into a 24-cup silicone mini-muffin pan (see Tip 2).

6 Bake for 15 minutes, or until a toothpick inserted into the center comes out clean.

7 Let cool in the pan for 5 minutes, then transfer the muffins to a wire rack to finish cooling. Let cool completely before serving.

Storage

Store in an airtight container in the refrigerator for up to 5 days. To freeze, store in a freezer-safe container for up to 2 months. To reheat, microwave for 15 to 20 seconds, until warmed through.

Tips

1. Egg-free? Replace the egg with a flax egg (see page 55).

2. If you don't have a silicone mini-muffin pan, you can use a metal 24-cup mini-muffin pan. If using a metal mini-muffin pan, be sure to grease the pan with butter or oil so the muffins won't stick.

Crispy Fish Sticks

prep **8 minutes** / cook **10 minutes** / serves **2 adults & 1 child**

Cooking spray (olive or avocado oil)

12 ounces (340 g) cod or tilapia fillets (2 medium fillets)

¼ teaspoon sweet paprika

¼ teaspoon garlic powder

⅛ teaspoon black pepper

½ cup (48 g) panko breadcrumbs

¼ cup (25 g) grated Parmesan

2 tablespoons all-purpose flour

1 egg (see Tip 1)

Fish is filled with omega-3 fatty acids, making it a great protein source for little ones. These fish sticks are crispy on the outside and moist and tender on the inside. They are great served with a dip or on their own! They're made quickly in the air fryer but can also be baked in the oven.

1 Spray an air fryer tray with cooking spray.

2 Slice the fillets into small strips about ½ inch (1 cm) thick. Season with paprika, garlic powder, and pepper.

3 Mix together the panko breadcrumbs, Parmesan, and flour in a shallow bowl.

4 Whisk the egg in a separate shallow bowl.

5 Dip each fillet strip into the breadcrumb mixture, shaking off any excess; dip into the egg mixture, shaking off any excess; and dip back into the breadcrumb mixture (see Tip 2). Place the battered strips on the air fryer tray, and repeat with the remaining strips.

6 Generously spray both sides of the fish sticks with cooking spray.

7 Air fry the sticks at 400°F (200°C) for 8 to 10 minutes, until golden brown (see Tip 3).

8 Serve warm or let cool.

Storage

Store cooled fish sticks in an airtight container in the fridge for up to 2 days. To freeze, store in a freezer-safe airtight container for up to 1 month. Reheat in the air fryer on the reheat setting.

Tips

1. Egg-free? Replace the egg with heavy cream or smooth, unsweetened yogurt.
2. The breadcrumb mixture may not stick well to the fish at first, but this "breadcrumb–egg–breadcrumb" mixture step will ensure that the egg mixture sticks.
3. No air fryer? You also can bake the fish sticks on a parchment paper–lined baking sheet in a 425°F (220°C) oven for 15 to 18 minutes, flipping halfway through, until golden brown.

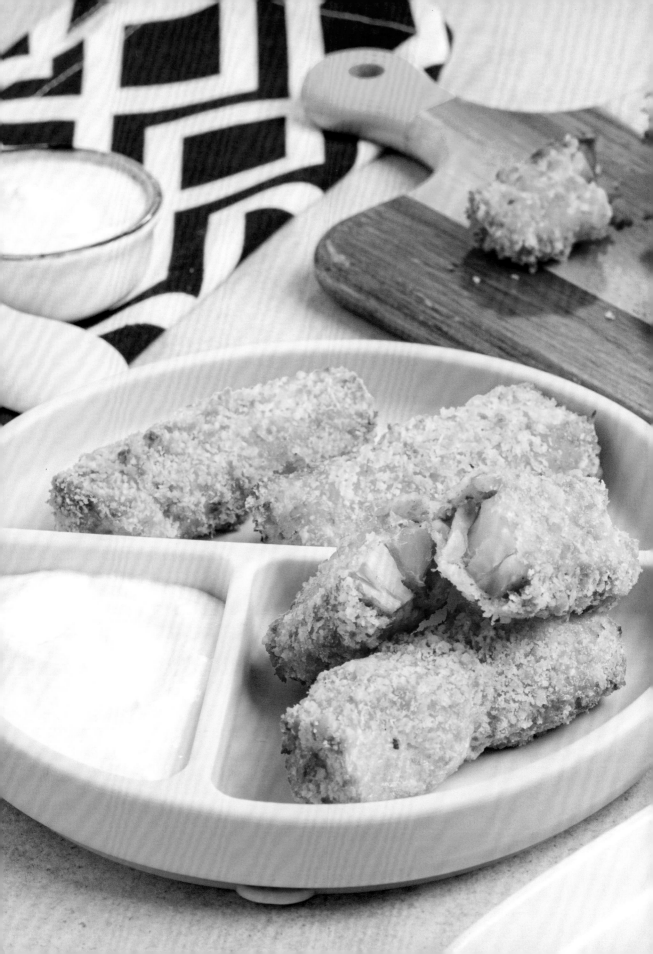

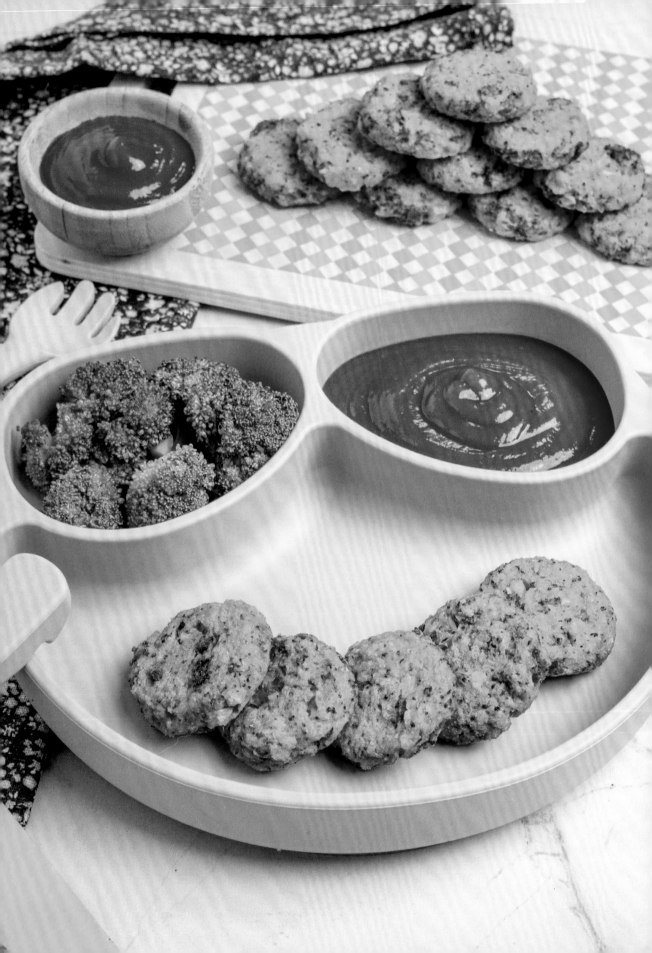

Sweet Potato Broccoli Bites

prep **15 minutes** / cook **20 minutes** / makes **20 bites**

Cooking spray (olive or avocado oil)

2 large sweet potatoes (about 1 pound/454 g)

1 cup (90 g) broccoli florets

¼ cup (24 g) panko breadcrumbs

¼ cup (25 g) grated Parmesan (see Tip 1)

½ teaspoon sweet paprika

½ teaspoon onion powder

These vegetable-packed bites are the perfect combination of savory and sweet. They are slightly crisp on the outside and soft and pillowy on the inside, so they're the ideal textures for little ones. Serve them on their own or with your favorite dip.

1 Preheat the oven to 400°F (200°C). Line a baking sheet with parchment paper, and spray with cooking spray.

2 Pierce the sweet potatoes several times with a fork, and microwave for 7 to 8 minutes, until tender and soft inside (see Tip 2). Scoop the flesh into a large bowl, and mash, leaving a little texture.

3 Place the broccoli florets in a microwave-safe bowl with 1 tablespoon of water and microwave for 3 minutes, or until fork-tender. (You can also steam the broccoli in a steamer basket for 10 minutes, or until tender.) Drain the liquid, and use kitchen scissors or a knife to finely chop the broccoli.

4 Add the broccoli, panko breadcrumbs, Parmesan, paprika, and onion powder to the bowl with the sweet potatoes. Use a fork to mix until well combined.

5 Scoop out tablespoon-sized portions of the mixture, and shape into small circles. Press down on the circles to flatten them into bites, and place them on the baking sheet. Lightly spray the bites with cooking spray (see Tip 3).

6 Bake for 20 minutes, or until golden.

7 Let cool completely on the baking sheet and then use a spatula to remove them from the pan. The bites will be soft at first but will firm up as they cool.

Storage

Store in an airtight container in the fridge for up to 4 days. To freeze, store in a freezer-safe container for up to 3 months. To reheat, microwave for 20 to 30 seconds, adding 10-second intervals as needed, until warmed through. You can also place on a baking sheet and reheat in a 350°F (180°C) oven for 10 minutes, or until warmed through.

Tips

1. Dairy-free? Swap the Parmesan with nutritional yeast.

2. You may also cook the sweet potatoes in the oven. Poke holes in the potatoes, and bake in a 425°F (220°C) oven for 45 to 50 minutes, until tender. If you have precooked sweet potatoes on hand, measure out 2 cups (480 g) of sweet potato flesh for this recipe.

3. If you prefer a crispier outer coating, dip the bites into some panko breadcrumbs after flattening them for added crunch!

Mini Pizza Calzones

prep **15 minutes** / cook **15 minutes** / makes **12 mini calzones**

1¾ cups (228 g) all-purpose flour

1 cup (240 g) plain whole milk Greek yogurt

1 tablespoon baking powder

½ teaspoon salt

½ cup (125 g) marinara sauce

½ cup (30 g) spinach, tightly packed, finely chopped

1 cup (113 g) shredded mozzarella

Cooking spray (olive or avocado oil)

The first time I served my eldest son pizza, I offered him half a slice. I'm not sure why I thought he wouldn't have trouble eating it, but I watched him struggle with it as a big glob of cheese dropped to the floor. His face was covered in sauce, the toppings were everywhere, and he barely got anything in his mouth. These mini pizza calzones are a manageable way for your little one to enjoy the taste of pizza without the mess. They store and reheat well for later use, and you can customize the fillings.

1 Preheat the oven to 425°F (220°C). Line a baking sheet with parchment paper.

2 Combine the flour, yogurt, baking powder, and salt in a medium bowl. Mix and knead until a dough comes together, then split into two equal pieces.

3 Dust a work surface with flour. Roll out the first piece into a ¼-inch-thick (6 mm) rectangle, and cut out four circles about 5 inches (13 cm) in diameter. Combine the scraps and roll them out again to get another two circles. Repeat this with the other half of the dough to get six more circles.

4 Spoon about 2 teaspoons of marinara sauce on half of each circle, leaving some space at the edge.

5 Sprinkle about 1 teaspoon of spinach on top of the sauce, then top with 1 heaping tablespoon mozzarella.

6 Fold the dough over the filling into a semicircle, and press down on the edges. Roll up the sides, and press over to seal closed. Place the mini calzones on the baking sheet.

7 Use a fork to poke a few holes at the top of each mini calzone. Spray the calzones with cooking spray.

8 Bake for 10 to 15 minutes, until golden.

9 Let cool completely before serving.

Storage

Store in an airtight container in the fridge for up to 3 days. To freeze, store in a freezer-safe airtight container for up to 2 months. To reheat, microwave for 20 to 30 seconds, adding 10-second intervals as needed, until warmed through. You can also place on a baking sheet and reheat in a 350°F (180°C) oven for 10 minutes, or until warmed through.

Tip

· Customize the calzone filling by using your favorite pizza toppings! Finely chop each topping, and be sure not to overstuff the calzones so you can still close them.

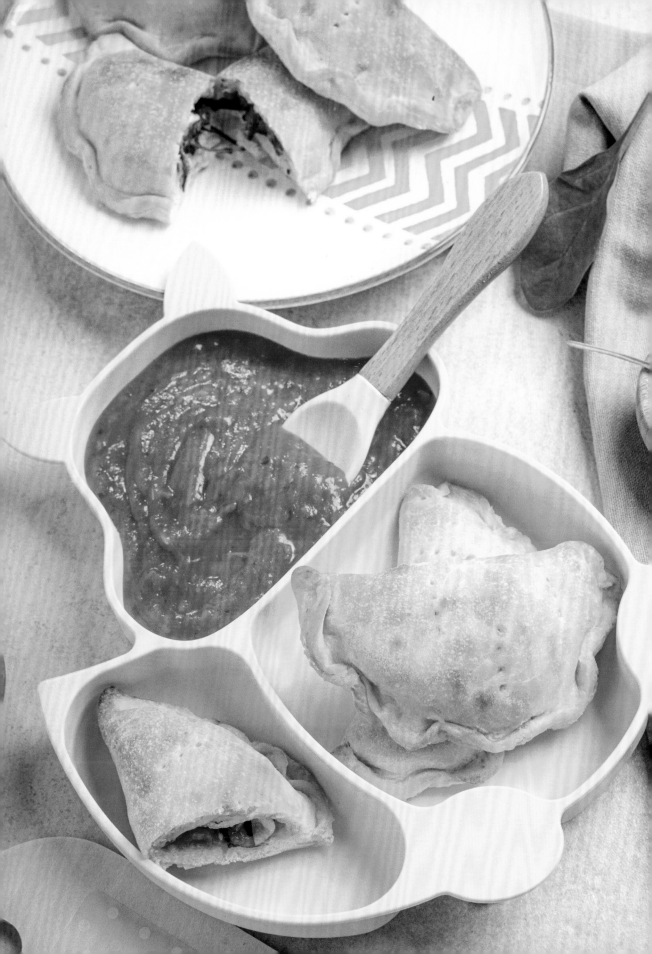

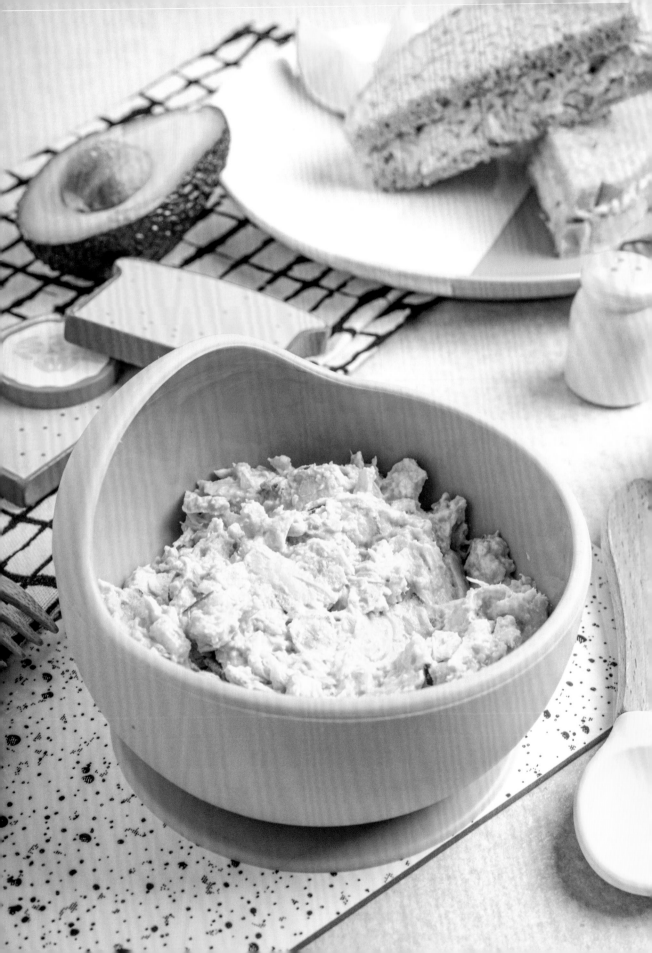

Avocado Chicken Salad

prep **5 minutes** / serves **1 adult & 1 child**

½ ripe avocado, pitted

2 tablespoons plain whole milk Greek yogurt (see Tip 1)

1 cup (125 g) shredded cooked chicken

2 tablespoons finely chopped red onion

¼ teaspoon garlic powder

Lime wedge

Sliced bread (optional)

Salt, to taste (optional, see Tip 2)

Avocados are loaded with healthy fats and nutrients. This chicken salad uses them as a base for a creamy, velvety texture. Enjoy this chicken salad cold or warm, as is or with a slice of toast. It's a great way to use leftover chicken breast!

1 Scoop the avocado flesh into a large bowl. Mash with a fork until smooth, leaving a few chunks if desired.

2 Add the yogurt, and mix to combine.

3 Add the chicken, onion, garlic powder, and juice of the lime wedge, and mix until combined.

4 Serve over sliced bread (if using) or as is!

Storage

This salad is best served fresh, but the lime juice will help prevent the avocado from browning too quickly. You can store it in an airtight container in the fridge for 1 day.

Tips

1. Dairy-free? Replace the Greek yogurt with unsweetened dairy-free yogurt.

2. Remove baby's portion, and add salt to taste for the rest of the family.

Oven-Baked Zucchini Tots

prep **10 minutes** / cook **20 minutes** / makes **15 to 18 tots**

2 cups (440 g) packed finely grated zucchini (from about 2 large zucchini, see Tip 1)

1 egg (see Tip 2)

½ cup (48 g) panko breadcrumbs

½ cup (50 g) grated Parmesan (see Tip 3)

¼ teaspoon garlic powder

¼ teaspoon onion powder

¼ teaspoon salt (optional)

These zucchini tots are soft-textured and perfect for babies and toddlers. They are packed with nutrients from the zucchini and make for a great, mess-free lunch. They're a fun take on traditional potato tots and an easy way of incorporating more veggies into your little one's diet.

1 Preheat the oven to 400°F (200°C). Line a baking sheet with parchment paper.

2 Use a cheesecloth, a clean kitchen towel, or your hands to squeeze out as much moisture from the zucchini as possible. You should end up with about 1 packed cup (about 180 g) of shredded zucchini. Transfer to a medium bowl.

3 Add the egg, panko breadcrumbs, Parmesan, garlic powder, onion powder, and salt (if using), and mix well to combine.

4 Scoop out tablespoon-sized portions, and shape them into small tots. Place the tots in the baking pan.

5 Bake for about 20 minutes, or until the edges of the tots begin to brown slightly. Shake the pan halfway through for even browning.

6 Let cool before serving.

Storage

Store in an airtight container in the fridge for up to 3 days. To freeze, store in a freezer-safe bag with most of the air removed for up to 3 months. To reheat, microwave for 20 to 30 seconds, adding 10-second intervals as needed, until warmed through. You can also place on a baking sheet and reheat in a 350°F (180°C) oven for 10 minutes, or until warmed through.

Tips

1. Use a cheese grater to grate the zucchini. Use the smallest holes for a smoother texture. You can leave on the skin for more nutrients.
2. Egg-free? Replace the egg with a flax egg (see page 55).
3. Mozzarella is a good low-sodium cheese option for babies.

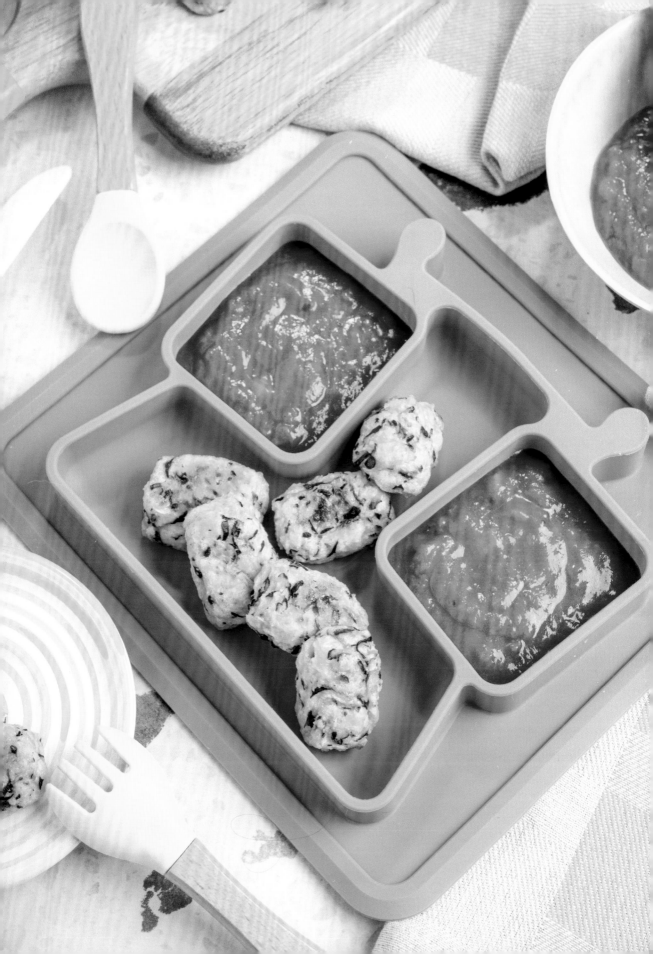

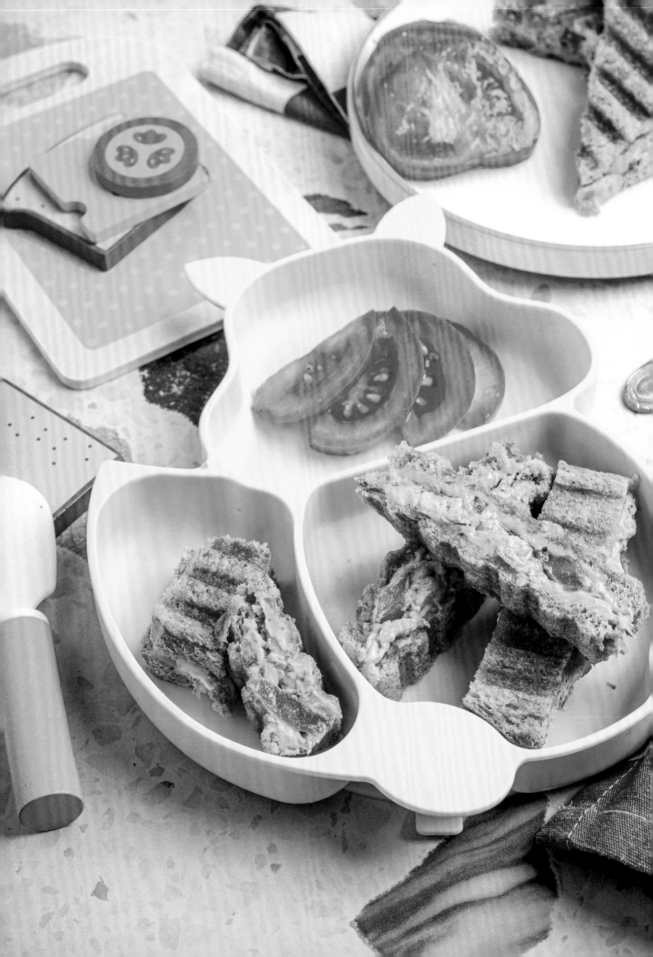

Tuna Melt Toasties

prep **5 minutes** / cook **5 minutes** / makes **2 sandwiches**

One 5-ounce (142 g) can tuna in water, drained (see Tip 1)

2 tablespoons plain whole milk Greek yogurt

1 to 2 tablespoons finely chopped red onion

2 tablespoons unsalted butter, softened

4 slices whole-wheat sandwich bread

4 slices cheddar

½ small Roma tomato, sliced

This tuna melt is the ultimate satisfying sandwich. It is oozing with melted cheese, sliced tomatoes, and tuna salad, all toasted together in a savory melt. It's a fun twist on a normal lunch sandwich that everyone in the family can enjoy!

1   Preheat a panini press or medium frying pan over medium-low heat.

2   Mix the tuna, yogurt, and onion in a small bowl.

3   Butter one side of each slice of bread, and place two slices of the bread into the pan, buttered side down.

4   Place one slice of cheddar onto each of two slices of bread and then place half of the tuna mixture on top of each slice. Add two to three slices of tomato, then top with an additional slice of cheese. Close the sandwich, buttered side up.

5   Cook the sandwiches on a panini press for 3 to 4 minutes or in a frying pan until golden on both sides, about 2 minutes per side. Press down on the sandwiches as they cook so the cheese melts.

6   Serve warm (see Tip 2).

Storage

These tuna melts are best served fresh, but you can prepare the tuna mixture in advance and store it in the fridge for up to 2 days. When ready to serve, simply add it to the sandwiches to cook.

Tips

1. Tuna is high in mercury and is recommended to be avoided (or offered in moderation) for children under the age of two. Canned salmon is a good alternative.
2. Slice the sandwich into strips to make it easier for baby to hold.

Mixed-Veggie Fritters

prep **10 minutes** / cook **6 minutes** / makes **15 to 18 mini fritters**

1 cup (220 g) packed finely grated zucchini (from about 1 large zucchini; see Tip 1)

½ cup (110 g) packed finely grated carrots (from about 1 medium carrot)

½ cup (84 g) corn kernels (see Tip 2)

¼ cup (33 g) all-purpose flour

¼ teaspoon garlic powder

¼ teaspoon onion powder

¼ teaspoon salt (optional)

1 egg (see Tip 3)

2 to 3 tablespoons mild-tasting oil

These fritters are one of my favorite ways to use up leftover veggies in the fridge. They're simple to make and so versatile. My go-to combination is zucchini, carrots, and corn, but you can customize these fritters with any veggies you have on hand! The vegetables soften inside the fritters as they cook, and they get a nice crisp coating on the outside. Serve with your favorite dip and veggies on the side!

1 Use a cheesecloth, a clean kitchen towel, or your hands to squeeze out as much moisture from the zucchini and carrots as possible.

2 Add the squeezed veggies to a bowl along with the corn.

3 Add the flour, garlic powder, onion powder, salt (if using), and egg, and mix until well combined.

4 Heat the oil in a large frying pan over medium heat. Working in batches, use a small cookie scoop to scoop small portions of the mixture (about 1 heaping tablespoon each) into the pan. Press down to flatten the fritters, and cook until golden on both sides, 2 to 3 minutes per side.

5 Transfer the cooked fritters to a paper towel–lined plate to cool, and repeat with the remaining mixture.

Storage

Store in an airtight container in the fridge for up to 3 days. To freeze, store in a freezer-safe bag with most of the air removed for up to 3 months. To reheat, microwave for 20 to 30 seconds, adding 10-second intervals as needed, until warmed through. You may also place on a baking sheet and reheat in a 350°F (180°C) oven for 10 minutes, or until warmed through.

Tips

1. Use a cheese grater to grate the zucchini. Use the smallest holes for a smoother texture. You can leave on the skin for more nutrients.
2. If you are preparing these for a baby under age one, smash the corn kernels before adding them to the bowl.
3. Egg-free? Replace the egg with a flax egg (see page 55).

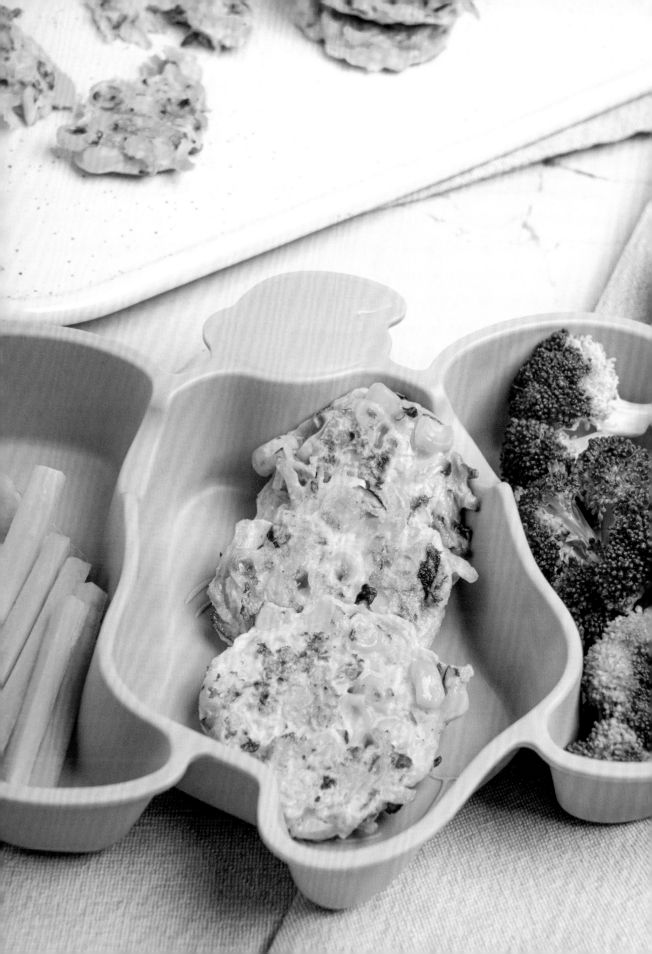

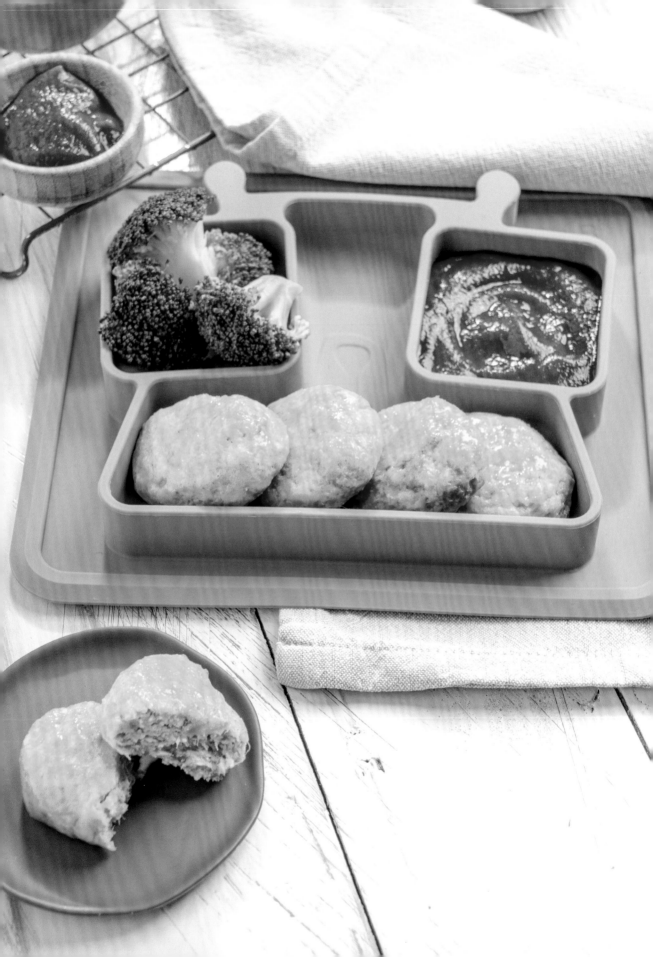

Sweet Potato Chicken Nuggets

prep **15 minutes** / cook **25 minutes** / makes **30 to 40 nuggets**

1 pound (454 g) ground chicken

1⅓ cups (320 g) mashed cooked sweet potato (see Tip 1)

¼ cup (24 g) panko breadcrumbs

1 tablespoon chili powder

2 teaspoons onion powder

1 teaspoon garlic powder

1 teaspoon sweet paprika

1 teaspoon salt (optional)

Cooking spray (olive or avocado oil)

If you've been on the hunt for a great-tasting, homemade chicken nugget recipe, the search ends here. These chicken nuggets are made with sweet potato as the base, which may sound strange, but trust me, it works! The sweet potato adds the perfect touch of sweetness to the nuggets, and the seasonings bring out the savory flavors. Everything comes together in one bowl, and I promise you won't be able to stop snacking on them!

1 Preheat the oven to 350°F (180°C). Line a baking sheet with parchment paper.

2 Add the chicken, sweet potato, panko breadcrumbs, chili powder, onion powder, garlic powder, paprika, and salt (if using) to a large bowl, and mix until well combined.

3 Wet your hands, then scoop out tablespoon-sized portions of the mixture and form them into nuggets (see Tip 2). Place the nuggets into the baking pan. Spray the nuggets with cooking spray.

4 Bake for 20 to 25 minutes, flipping halfway through, until golden.

5 Let cool completely before serving (see Tip 3).

Storage

Store in an airtight container in the fridge for up to 4 days. To freeze, store in a freezer-safe airtight container for up to 3 months. To reheat, microwave for 20 to 30 seconds, adding 10-second intervals as needed, until warmed through. You can also place on a baking sheet and reheat in a 350°F (180°C) oven for 10 minutes, or until warmed through.

Tips

1. You can precook sweet potatoes in the oven (poke holes in the potatoes, and bake at 425°F/220°C for 45 to 50 minutes, until tender) or in the microwave (poke holes in the potatoes, and microwave for 5 to 6 minutes, until tender). Let the potatoes cool, then peel and mash them.

2. It's very important to wet your hands and keep them moist as you shape the nuggets because ground chicken tends to be very sticky. The water will make it easier to scoop and shape the nuggets. If you prefer a crispier coating, dip the nuggets into extra panko breadcrumbs before placing them on the baking sheet.

3. If your little one has developed the pincer grasp, dice the nuggets into small pieces so that they can practice picking up items with their index finger and thumb.

Cheesy Carrot Balls

prep **10 minutes** / cook **15 minutes** / makes **10 bites**

1 cup (220 g) packed finely grated carrots

⅓ cup (38 g) shredded cheddar

¼ cup (24 g) panko breadcrumbs

1 egg (see Tip 1)

¼ teaspoon garlic powder

¼ teaspoon onion powder

¼ teaspoon salt (optional)

¼ teaspoon black pepper (optional)

This is a signature Feeding Tiny Bellies recipe! These carrot balls are hands down my boys' favorite way of enjoying carrots. They were never big fans of carrots, so I wanted to come up with a new, fun way of serving them to get my boys excited about eating them. These bites are the perfect way to use up carrots in a bright, fun, orange-colored bite!

1 Preheat the oven to 400°F (200°C). Line a baking sheet with parchment paper.

2 Use a cheesecloth, a clean kitchen towel, or your hands to squeeze out as much moisture from the carrots as possible.

3 Add the carrots to a large bowl along with the cheddar, panko breadcrumbs, egg, garlic powder, onion powder, salt (if using), and pepper (if using). Mix well.

4 Scoop out tablespoon-sized portions of the mixture, and roll them into small balls. Place the balls into the baking pan (see Tip 2).

5 Bake for 15 minutes, or until the edges start to brown slightly.

6 Let cool before serving.

Storage

Store in an airtight container in the fridge for up to 3 days. To freeze, store in a freezer-safe bag with most of the air removed for up to 3 months. To reheat, microwave for 20 to 30 seconds, adding 10-second intervals as needed, until warmed through. You can also place on a baking sheet and reheat in a 350°F (180°C) oven for 10 minutes, or until warmed through.

Tips

1. Egg-free? Swap the egg with a flax egg (see page 55).
2. If serving to a young baby, quarter the bites. You may also press down on the balls before baking to form thin discs.
3. Double the recipe to make more carrot balls to freeze for easy lunches throughout the week!

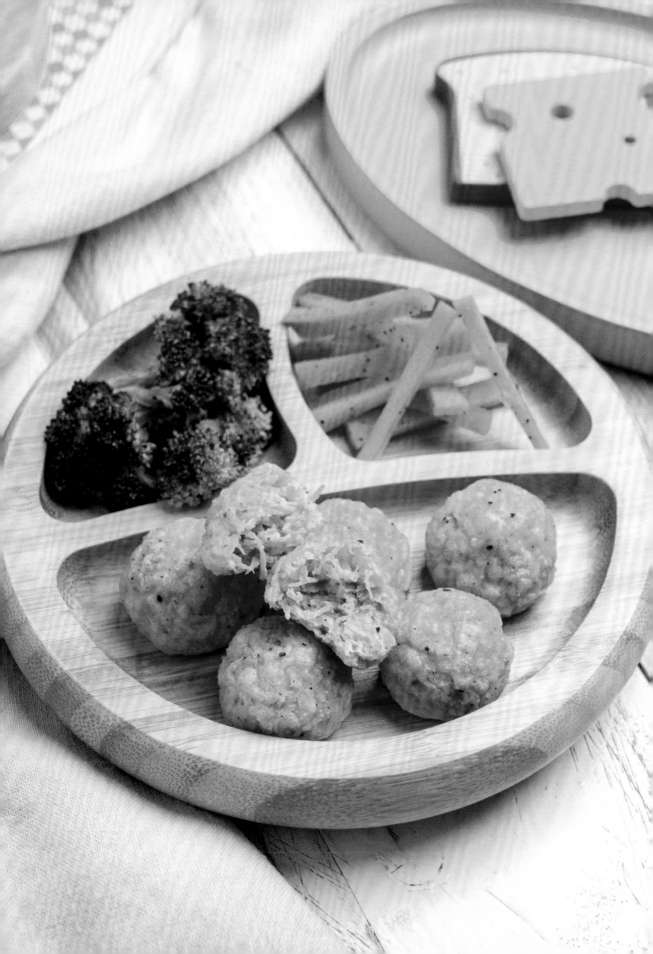

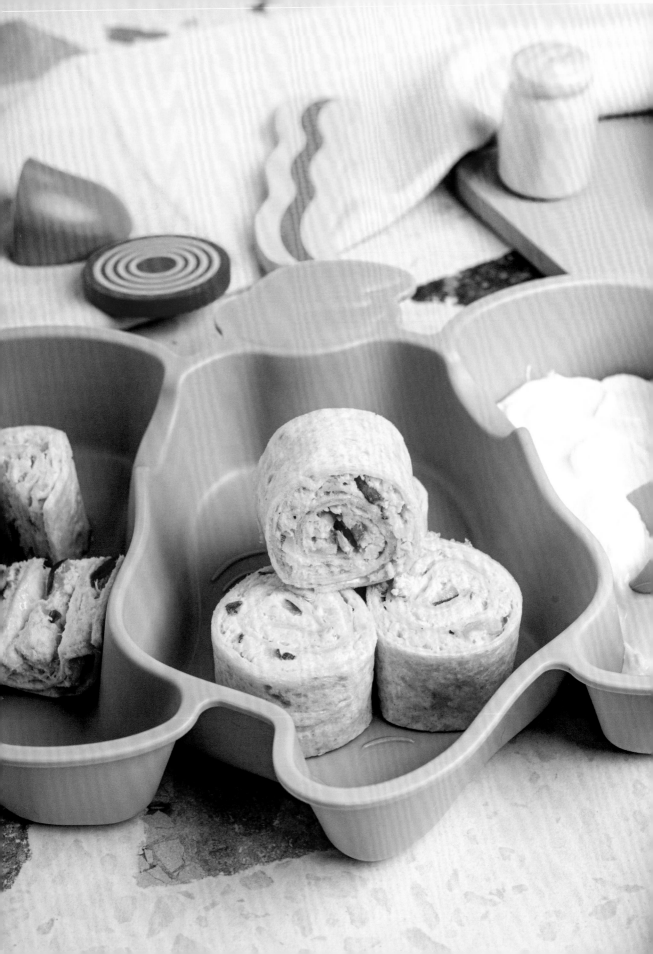

Salmon Salad Wraps

prep **5 minutes** / serves **1 adult & 1 child**

1 large cooked salmon
   fillet (about 6
   ounces/170 g; see Tip 1)
2 tablespoons plain
   whole milk Greek yogurt
   (see Tip 2)
2 tablespoons finely
   chopped red onion
⅛ teaspoon garlic
   powder
⅛ teaspoon salt (optional;
   see Tip 3)
Two 8-inch (20 cm) flour
   tortillas

These salmon pinwheel wraps are one of my favorite fun ways to use up leftover salmon fillets for a quick and easy lunch. The Greek yogurt brings a creaminess to the filling, and the red onion adds great texture and flavor.

1 Place the salmon in a bowl, and use a fork to flake and mash it. You'll have about ½ cup (170 g) mashed salmon.

2 Add the yogurt, onion, garlic powder, and salt (if using), and mix to combine.

3 Evenly divide the salmon mixture between the tortillas, and spread it out, leaving about 1 inch (2.5 cm) of space at one end of the tortilla to prevent the filling from coming out. Roll each tortilla into a tight log.

4 Slice the tortilla wraps into 1-inch (2.5 cm) pieces, and serve.

Storage

These salmon pinwheels are best served fresh but can be stored in an airtight container in the fridge for up to 2 days. Store the salmon mixture in a separate container, then spread it onto the tortillas right before you are ready to serve.

Tips

1. You may also use a 5-ounce (142 g) can of salmon in place of a cooked salmon fillet. Drain the excess liquid in the can before using.

2. Dairy-free? Replace the Greek yogurt with unsweetened dairy-free yogurt. If you prefer a creamier texture, stir in an extra tablespoon of yogurt.

3. Remove baby's portion of the salmon mixture, and add salt to taste for the rest of the family!

Veggie Pinwheels

prep **8 minutes** / cook **25 minutes** / makes **8 pinwheels**

1 sheet puff pastry (8.6 ounces/245 g), thawed

½ cup (110 g) packed finely grated zucchini

½ cup (110 g) packed finely grated carrots

½ cup (57 g) shredded cheddar (see Tips 1 and 2)

Cooking spray (olive or avocado oil)

These pinwheels are a fun way to enjoy some classic veggies! The tender flakiness of puff pastry pairs so well with the cheese and shredded veggies for a simple lunch option. Feel free to add extra veggies or leftover chicken for a super nutrient-dense meal.

1 Preheat the oven to 400°F (200°C). Line a baking sheet with parchment paper.

2 Dust a work surface with flour and then unfold the puff pastry sheet onto the surface.

3 Use a cheesecloth, a clean kitchen towel, or your hands to squeeze out as much moisture from the grated zucchini and carrots as possible. You should end up with about ¾ cup (about 90 g) of the veggie mixture. Sprinkle the veggies evenly over the puff pastry, then sprinkle the cheddar evenly on top.

4 Tightly roll the puff pastry into a log lengthwise, and slice it into eight equal pieces. Place the pinwheels on the baking sheet, and spray the pieces with cooking spray (see Tip 3). Leave around 1 to 2 inches (2.5 to 5 cm) of space between each of the pieces on the baking sheet because they will spread as they bake.

5 Bake for 20 to 25 minutes, until golden.

6 Let cool slightly before serving.

Storage

Store in an airtight container in the fridge for up to 3 days. To freeze, store in a freezer-safe bag with most of the air removed for up to 1 month. To reheat, place on a baking sheet, and bake in a 350°F (180°C) oven for 10 minutes, or until warmed through.

Tips

1. If preparing these for a baby, mozzarella is a good low-sodium cheese option.

2. Dairy-free? Swap the shredded cheese with dairy-free cheese shreds.

3. You can brush the top with a whisked egg instead of the cooking spray for a shiny, golden-brown crust.

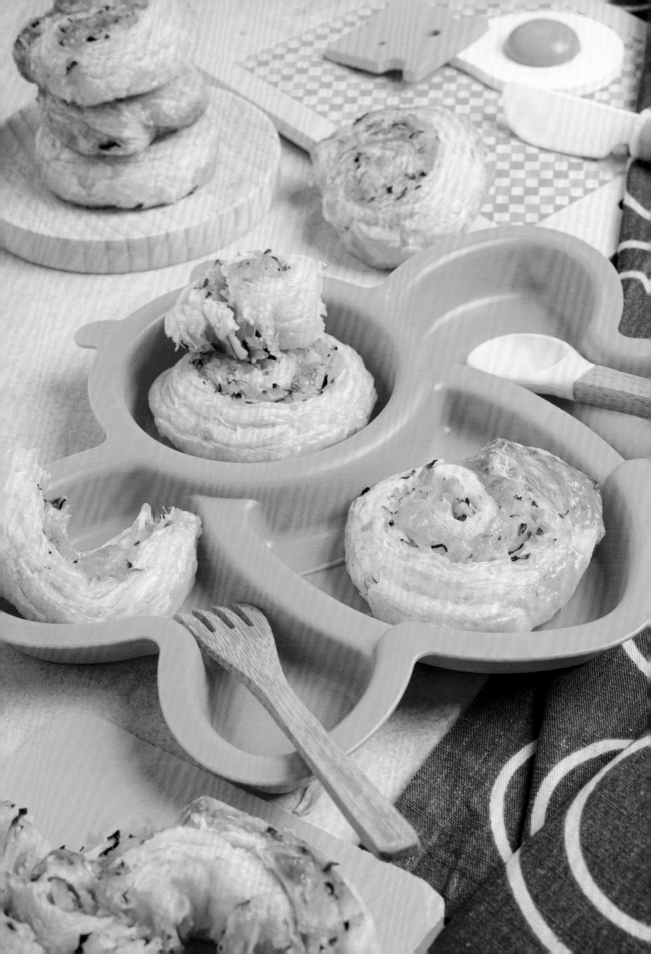

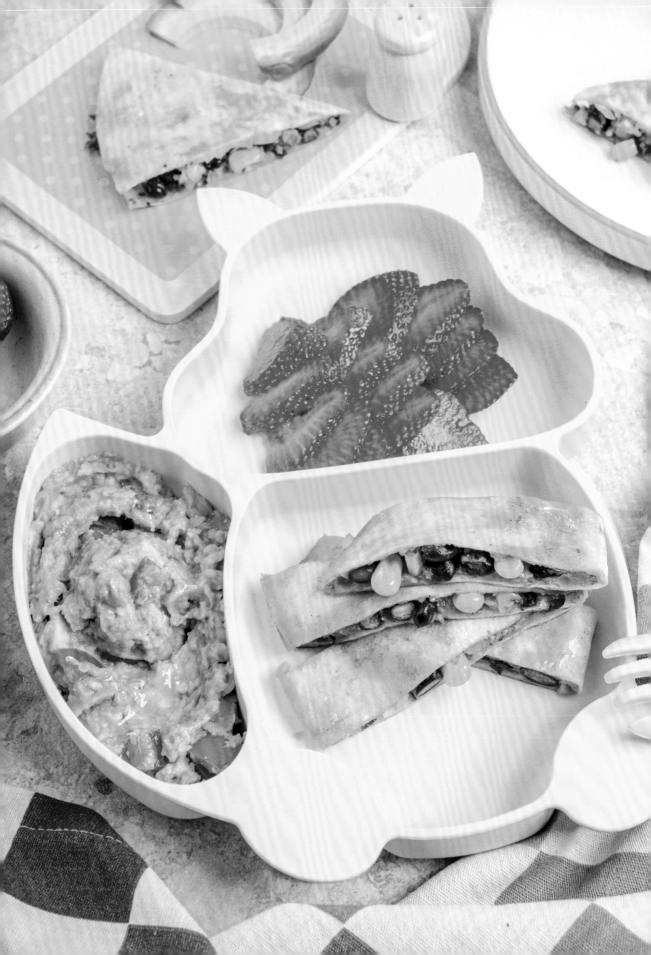

Bean & Corn Quesadillas

prep **8 minutes** / cook **5 minutes** / makes **2 quesadillas**

Seasoning Mixture

1 teaspoon chili powder

¼ teaspoon ground cumin

¼ teaspoon sweet paprika

⅛ teaspoon dried oregano

Quesadillas

½ cup (57 g) shredded cheddar (see Tip 1)

¼ cup (42 g) canned black beans, drained and rinsed

¼ cup (42 g) corn kernels

2 tablespoons finely diced red onion

Two 8-inch (20 cm) flour tortillas

1 tablespoon unsalted butter

These quesadillas are so filling yet so simple to make. The beans add great protein and fiber, and the corn adds a nice sweetness and crunch. Pair them with some salsa, sour cream, or guacamole for a quick, satisfying, Mexican-inspired lunch!

1 Make the seasoning mixture: Combine the chili powder, cumin, paprika, and oregano in a small bowl.

2 Make the quesadillas: Combine the cheddar, beans, corn, onion, and seasoning mixture in a medium bowl (see Tip 2).

3 Preheat a large frying pan over medium heat.

4 Place half of the filling mixture on one half of one tortilla, and fold the tortilla over the filling. Repeat with the remaining filling mixture and the second tortilla.

5 Add the butter to the pan to melt. Add the quesadillas, and cook until the quesadillas are golden on both sides and the cheese has fully melted, 2 to 3 minutes per side.

6 Slice into triangles or strips, and serve.

Storage

Store in an airtight container in the fridge for up to 2 days. To reheat, heat a skillet over low heat, and cook the quesadillas until warmed through, about 2 minutes per side.

Tips

1. If preparing these for a baby, mozzarella is a good low-sodium cheese option.

2. Feel free to add some shredded chicken or steak in the filling mixture for an extra iron source!

Spinach & Tomato Quesadillas

prep **8 minutes** / cook **5 minutes** / makes **2 quesadillas**

¼ cup (15 g) spinach, tightly packed

¾ cup (85 g) shredded mozzarella (see Tip 1)

½ cup (100 g) diced Roma tomatoes

Two 8-inch (20 cm) flour tortillas

1 tablespoon unsalted butter

I love the combination of tomatoes and melted cheese, and they pair so well together in these quesadillas. The spinach provides a great source of iron, and the tomatoes add vitamin C to help boost iron consumption!

1 Finely chop the spinach and set aside.

2 Preheat a large frying pan over medium heat.

3 Place half of the mozzarella, half of the tomatoes, and half of the spinach on one half of one tortilla, and fold the tortilla over the filling (see Tip 2). Repeat with the remaining filling mixture and the second tortilla.

4 Add the butter to the pan to melt. Add the quesadillas, and cook until the quesadillas are golden on both sides and the cheese has fully melted, 2 to 3 minutes per side.

5 Slice into triangles or strips, and serve.

Storage

Store in an airtight container in the fridge for up to 2 days. To reheat, heat a skillet over low heat, and cook the quesadillas until warmed through, about 2 minutes per side.

Tips

1. Dairy-free? Swap the mozzarella with dairy-free shreds.

2. Feel free to add some shredded chicken or steak to the filling mixture for an extra iron source!

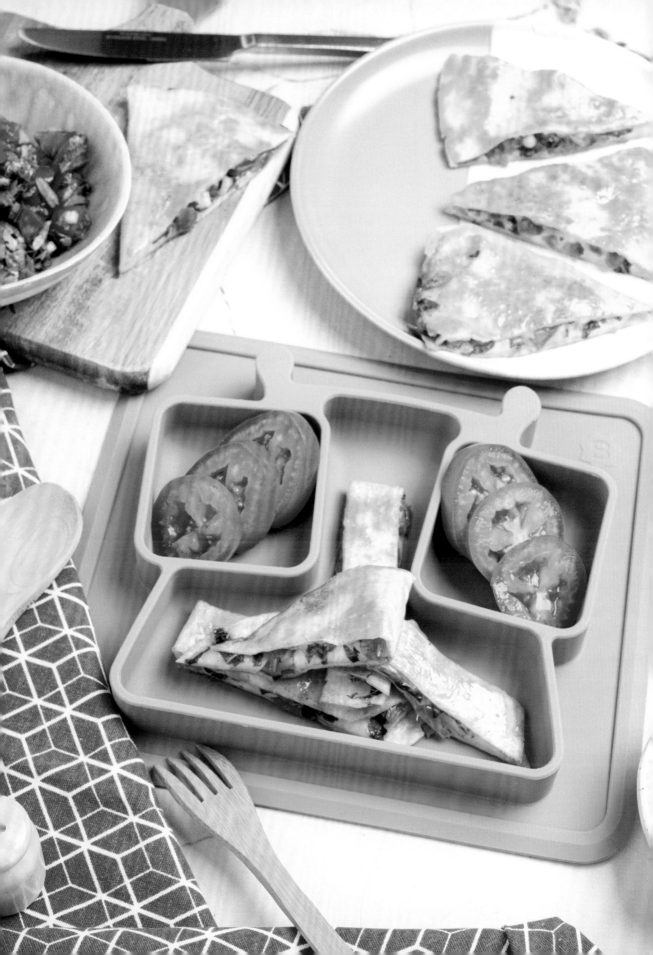

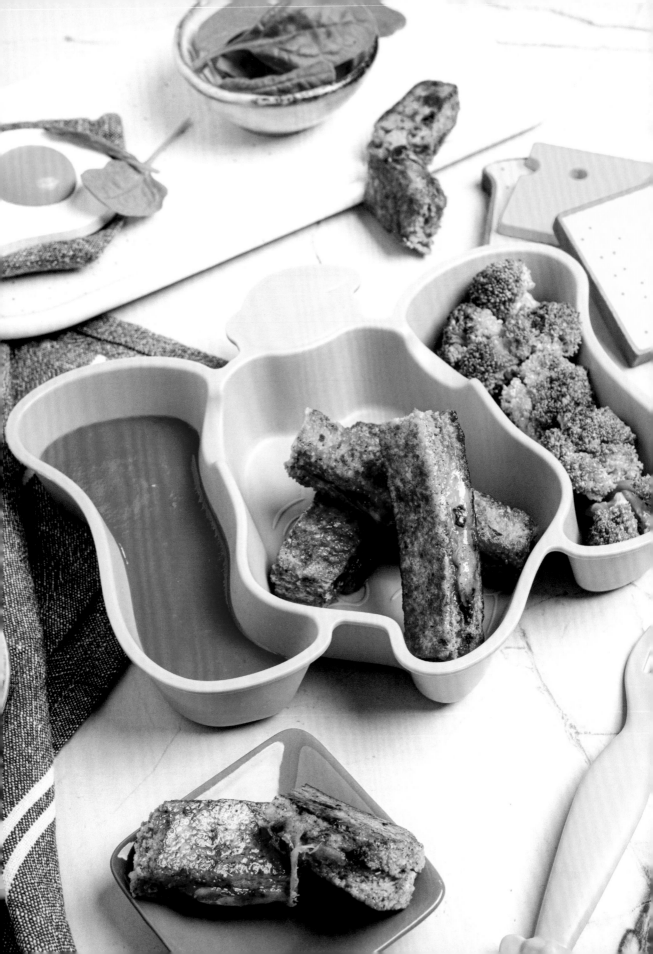

Pizza French Toast Sticks

prep **5 minutes** / cook **10 minutes** / serves **1 adult & 1 child**

4 slices whole-wheat bread

¼ cup (62 g) marinara sauce

¼ cup (28 g) shredded mozzarella (see Tip 1)

2 tablespoons finely chopped spinach

1 tablespoon unsalted butter

1 egg (see Tip 2)

2 tablespoons milk

¼ teaspoon Italian seasoning

This savory take on classic French toast is a fun, easy-to-make lunch option for the whole family. You can serve these sticks plain for a baby or with your favorite sauces for the rest of the family to dip into. I love dipping them into marinara sauce for that classic pizza flavor.

1 Remove the crusts from the bread, and evenly spread the marinara sauce onto two slices of bread.

2 Top each slice with equal parts mozzarella and spinach (see Tip 3). Place the remaining bread slices on top to form two sandwiches, and use a rolling pin or your hands to roll out or press down firmly on the sandwiches to seal them closed. Slice each sandwich into three to four sticks.

3 Heat a medium frying pan over medium heat, then add the butter to melt.

4 Whisk together the egg, milk, and Italian seasoning in a small bowl until combined. Dip each pizza stick into the egg mixture, shaking off any excess.

5 Cook the sticks until golden brown on all sides, about 2 minutes per side. Serve warm.

Storage

Store in an airtight container in the fridge for up to 3 days. To freeze, store in a freezer-safe bag with most of the air removed for up to 3 months. To reheat, microwave for 30 seconds, adding 10-second increments as needed, until warmed through.

Tips

1. Dairy-free? Swap the mozzarella with dairy-free shreds.
2. Egg-free? Spread a thick layer of butter on both sides of the outside of the sandwiches at the end of step 2 before cutting the sandwiches into sticks, skip step 4, and instead sprinkle the Italian seasoning on the buttered sandwiches. (Omit the milk.) Cook as directed in step 5.
3. Feel free to add other fillings like bell peppers, mushrooms, or pepperoni, all finely chopped.

Sweet Potato & Apple Fritters

prep **10 minutes** / cook **10 minutes** / makes **18 to 22 mini fritters**

1 cup (240 g) mashed
  cooked sweet potato
  (see Tip 1)

1 large apple (see Tip 2)

1 egg (see Tip 3)

¼ cup (33 g) all-purpose
  flour

½ teaspoon ground
  cinnamon

1 tablespoon unsalted
  butter

Sweet potatoes and apples pair so well together. The potatoes and apples combine to make sweet, soft-textured fritters that are great served warm or cold. The mixture comes together in one bowl and cooks quickly on the stove for little bites you won't be able to stop snacking on.

1 Place the mashed sweet potato in a large bowl.

2 Peel and grate the apple using the large hole side of a box grater, and add the shreds to the bowl. Mix the apple into the sweet potato until combined.

3 Add the egg, flour, and cinnamon to the bowl, and mix to combine.

4 Heat a large frying pan over medium-low heat, and add the butter to melt.

5 Working in batches, scoop tablespoon-sized portions of the sweet potato–apple mixture into the pan. Press down gently to flatten each fritter.

6 Cook until golden brown, 2 minutes per side. Transfer to a paper towel–lined plate, and repeat with the remaining mixture.

7 Let cool before serving. They will seem soft at first but will firm up as they cool.

Storage

Store in an airtight container in the fridge for up to 3 days. To freeze, store in a freezer-safe bag with most of the air removed for up to 3 months. To reheat, microwave for 20 to 30 seconds, adding 10-second intervals as needed, until warmed through. You can also place on a baking sheet and reheat in a 350°F (180°C) oven for 10 minutes, or until warmed through.

Tips

1. You may precook sweet potatoes in the oven (poke holes in the potatoes, and bake at 425°F/220°C for 45 to 50 minutes, until tender) or in the microwave (poke holes in the potatoes, and microwave for 5 to 6 minutes, until tender). Let the potatoes cool, then peel and mash them.

2. Honeycrisp and Fuji apples are my favorite varieties to use for this recipe, but any sweet apple will work!

3. Egg-free? Swap the egg with a flax egg (see page 55).

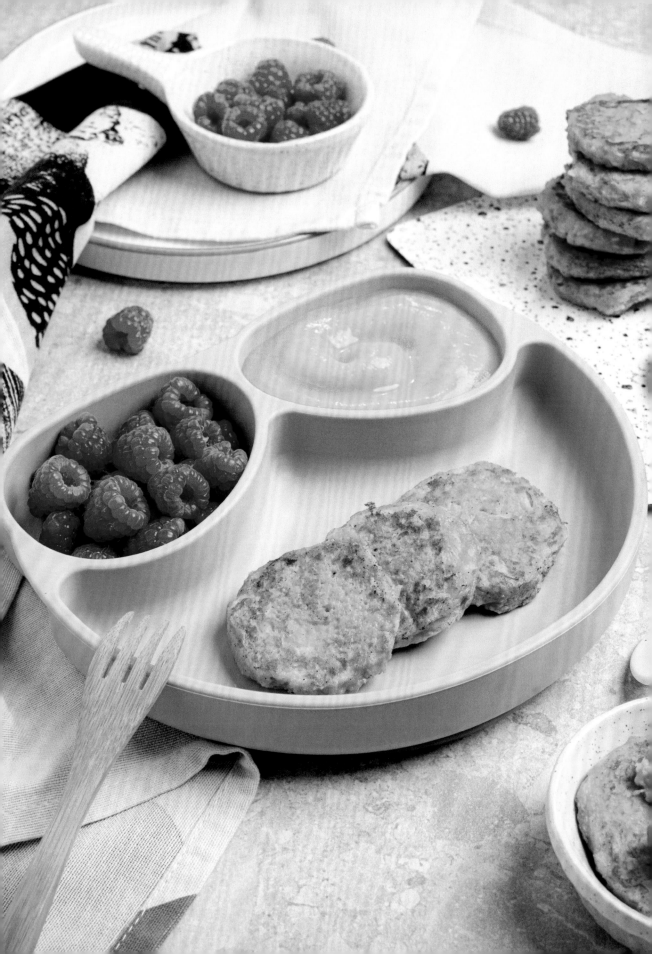

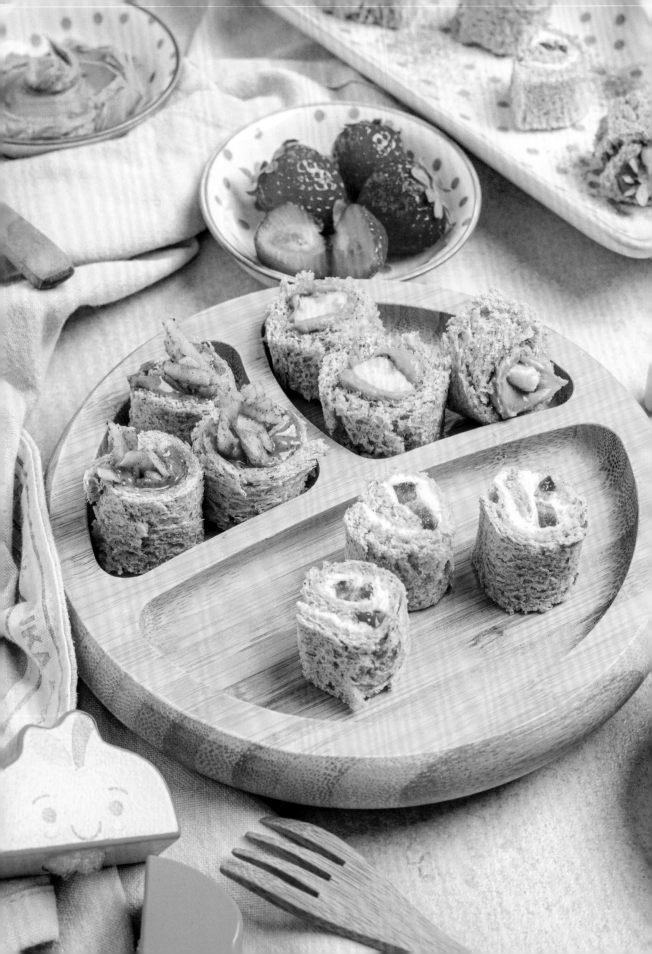

Fruity "Sushi" Rolls

prep **5 minutes** / serves **1 adult & 1 child**

These fruity "sushi" rolls are a go-to lunch option for busy days. I love that they're simple, don't require any cooking, and are still rich in protein! Okay, so they have nothing to do with actual sushi, besides the fact that they're rolled and sliced, but they definitely make serving a classic sandwich more fun!

1 Remove the crusts from the slices of bread, and use a rolling pin to thinly flatten the bread slices.

2 Spread 1 tablespoon of spread (peanut butter, almond butter, or cream cheese for your preferred flavor) on one side of each slice of bread.

3 Place the fruit (banana, apple, or strawberries) in a line on the long end of the bread. Sprinkle the cinnamon over the fruit.

4 Starting with the fruit on the bottom, roll the bread over the filling into a tight log (see Tip 2).

5 Use a sharp knife to slice the log into 1-inch-thick (2.5 cm) pieces.

DF EF V

Peanut Butter Banana "Sushi" Rolls

3 slices whole-wheat bread

3 tablespoons natural peanut butter

½ medium ripe banana, peeled and split into thirds (see Tip 1)

¼ teaspoon ground cinnamon

DF EF V

Almond Butter Apple "Sushi" Rolls

3 slices whole-wheat bread

3 tablespoons natural almond butter

1 apple, grated and lightly squeezed (preferably Honeycrisp)

¼ teaspoon ground cinnamon

EF NF V

Strawberry Cheesecake "Sushi" Rolls

3 slices whole-wheat bread

3 tablespoons cream cheese

2 large strawberries, diced

¼ teaspoon ground cinnamon

Storage

These rolls are best served fresh. To make them in advance, wrap the sandwich log tightly in plastic wrap, but don't slice until you're ready to serve. The unsliced log will keep fresh in the fridge for up to 2 days.

Tips

1. Use your finger to split the banana into natural thirds. Alternatively, you can roll up half of a banana.

2. Sprinkle some hemp hearts or flaxseeds on top of the "sushi" pieces for an added nutritional boost!

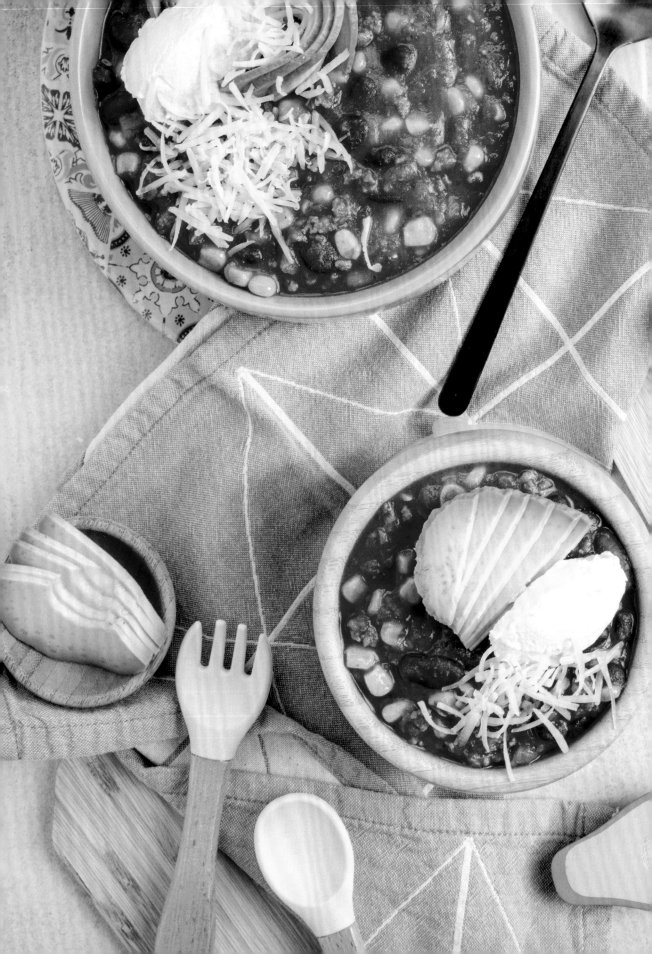

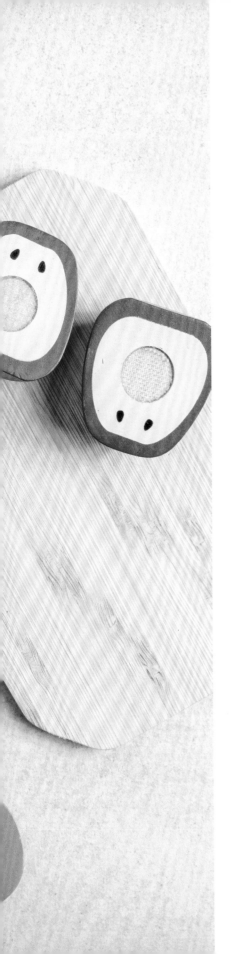

Dinner

Dinner recipes are often the most stressful to prepare, but I'm here to tell you that it doesn't have to be that way! Dinnertime doesn't have to be a production, nor does it have to be complicated. Whether you love cooking or not, you don't have to spend hours in the kitchen to prepare a meal for the whole family. This chapter is full of simple recipes that are flavorful and filling. From sheet pan bakes to one-pot pastas, I share some fun options that I hope will become some of your family's go-to meals!

Chicken & Broccoli Meatballs

prep **10 minutes** / cook **20 minutes** / makes **28 to 30 meatballs**

2½ cups (225 g) broccoli florets (see Tip 1)

1 pound (454 g) ground chicken

½ cup (48 g) panko breadcrumbs

½ cup (50 g) grated Parmesan

1 egg (see Tip 2)

½ teaspoon onion powder

½ teaspoon salt

⅛ teaspoon black pepper

Cooking spray (olive or avocado oil)

I'm always looking for fun new ways to incorporate broccoli into recipes, and these meatballs do not disappoint! Whenever I make them, I have to stop myself from eating the entire batch before I realize that we haven't had dinner yet. They are so good as a snack on their own or simmered in a marinara sauce. This is definitely a go-to recipe in our home, and I hope it will become a staple in yours as well!

1 Preheat the oven to 400°F (200°C). Line a baking sheet with parchment paper.

2 Place the broccoli florets in a microwave-safe bowl with 1 tablespoon of water, and microwave for 3 minutes, or until fork-tender. (You may also steam the broccoli in a steamer basket for 10 minutes, or until tender.)

3 Drain the liquid, and use kitchen scissors or a knife to finely chop the broccoli. (You may also quickly pulse the broccoli in a blender if you prefer a finer texture.) You should have about 1½ cups (135 g) of finely chopped broccoli.

4 Add the broccoli, chicken, panko breadcrumbs, Parmesan, egg, onion powder, salt, and pepper to a large bowl, and mix to combine. (Do not overmix because overmixing can cause the meat to become tough when baked.)

5 Scoop out tablespoon-sized portions of the mixture, and roll them into small balls (see Tip 3). Place the balls onto the baking sheet, and spray them with cooking spray.

6 Bake for 18 to 22 minutes, until cooked through. The meatballs are fully cooked when an instant-read thermometer inserted into the center of a meatball reads 165°F (75°C).

Storage

Store in an airtight container in the fridge for up to 3 days. To freeze, arrange the meatballs in a single layer on a baking sheet, and freeze until solid. Transfer the meatballs to a freezer-safe bag with most of the air removed, and freeze for up to 2 months. To reheat, place on a baking sheet, cover with foil, and bake in a 300°F (150°C) oven for 15 minutes, or until warmed through.

Tips

1. Swap the broccoli with different veggies for some other flavor variations!
2. Egg-free? Replace the egg with a flax egg (see page 55).
3. If serving this to a baby, quarter the meatballs. You may also make jumbo-sized meatballs (bigger than baby's fist).

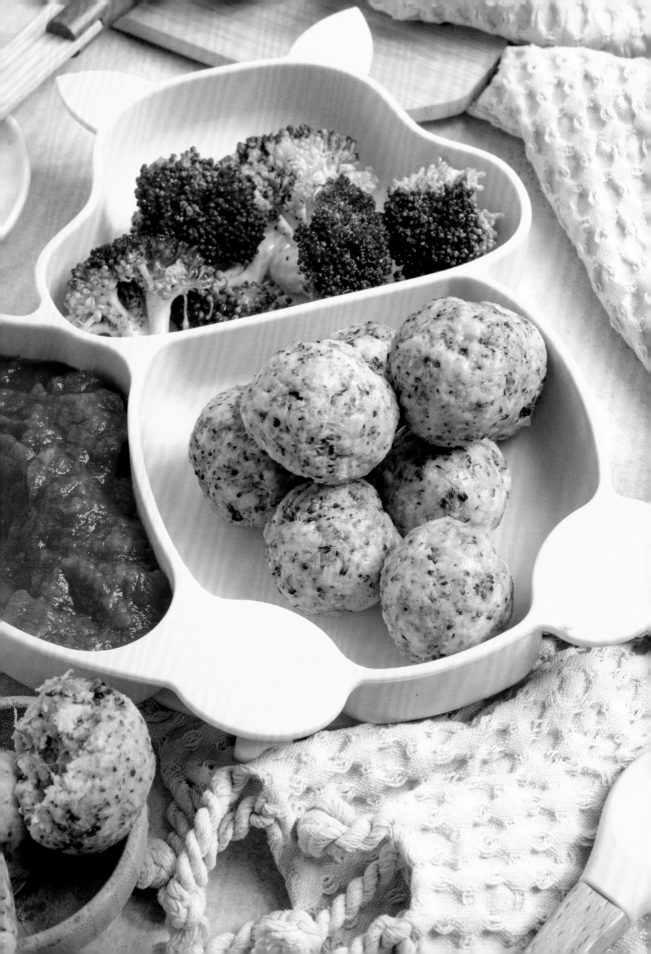

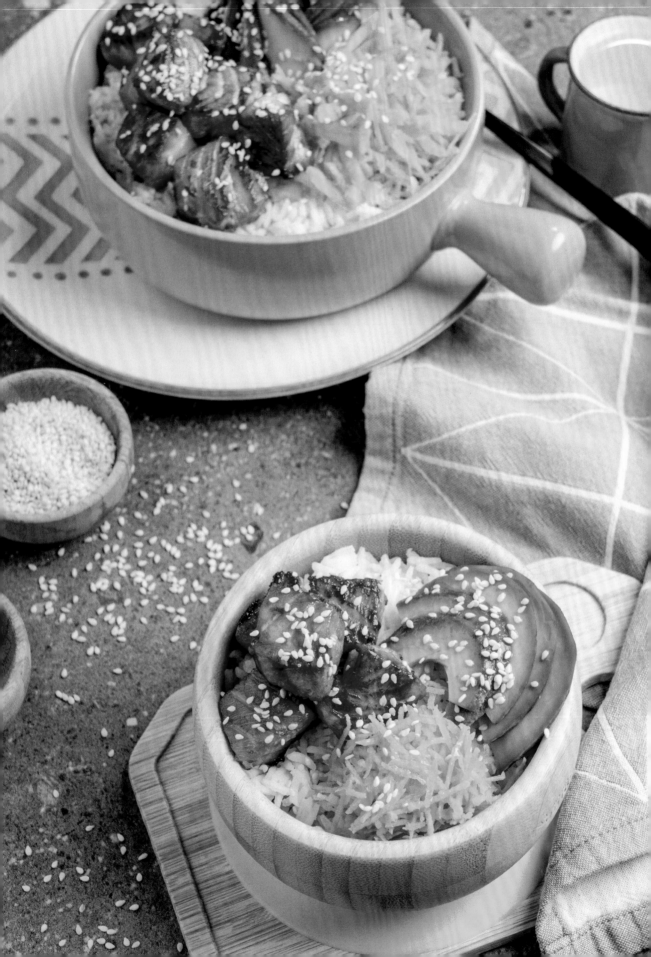

Maple-glazed Salmon Rice Bowls

prep **25 minutes** / cook **5 minutes** / serves **1 adult & 2 children**

2 salmon fillets (5 to 6 ounces/142 to 170 g each; see Tip 1)

3 tablespoons low-sodium soy sauce

3 tablespoons maple syrup

1 teaspoon minced fresh ginger

¼ teaspoon garlic powder

2 tablespoons olive oil, divided

For Serving

2 cups (400 g) cooked white rice

1 avocado, peeled, pitted, and sliced

½ cup (110 g) finely shredded carrots

Sesame seeds (optional)

If you're a fan of sweet and savory flavors, you'll love this maple-glazed salmon. The salmon is marinated in a simple five-ingredient marinade, lightly pan-fried, and served over rice. The sweet glaze pairs perfectly with the flaky fish for an Asian-inspired bowl the whole family will love!

1 Slice the salmon into 1-inch (2.5 cm) cubes (see Tip 2).

2 Mix the soy sauce, maple syrup, ginger, garlic powder, and 1 tablespoon of oil in a large bowl or container. Add the salmon, and turn to coat in the marinade. Let marinate for at least 20 minutes at room temperature or for up to 1 hour in the refrigerator.

3 Heat the remaining 1 tablespoon of oil in a medium nonstick pan over medium heat. Remove the salmon from the marinade, reserving the marinade (see Tip 3). Add the salmon to the pan, and cook until opaque, 2 to 3 minutes on one side, then flip and cook the other side until golden on all edges, 1 to 2 minutes more (see Tip 4).

4 Serve over white rice, and top with avocado, shredded carrots, and sesame seeds (if using).

Storage

Store in an airtight container in the fridge for up to 3 days. Reheat in a skillet over medium heat until warmed through, 1 to 2 minutes per side.

Tips

1. Press the salmon fillets firmly to check for bones before using.

2. If preparing this for a baby, you can set aside a few pieces of salmon to cook without the marinade and assemble their bowl separately.

3. If you would like to safely use the remaining fish marinade as a sauce, pour it into a saucepan over medium-high heat, bring it to a complete boil, and cook until the temperature reaches 165°F (75°C), about 5 minutes. Remove from the heat, and let cool. This will ensure that all the bacteria have been killed and the marinade is safe to eat.

4. Prefer to bake? Bake the salmon at 400°F (200°C) for 12 to 15 minutes, until opaque and golden on all edges.

Sweet Potato Tuna Patties

prep **20 minutes** / cook **8 minutes** / makes **8 patties**

1 cup (240 g) mashed cooked sweet potato (see Tip 1)

Two 5-ounce (142 g) cans tuna in water, drained (see Tip 2)

½ cup (48 g) panko breadcrumbs

¼ cup (35 g) finely diced red onion

1 egg (see Tip 3)

½ teaspoon salt (optional)

¼ teaspoon garlic powder

Mild-tasting oil, for frying

Creamy sweet potato blends with tuna to form these irresistible mini cakes, which are slightly crispy on the outside and tender on the inside. Even non–fish lovers will enjoy them! They can be eaten in a sandwich, with a dip, or as is.

1 Add the sweet potato, tuna, panko breadcrumbs, onion, egg, salt (if using), and garlic powder to a bowl, and mix until well combined.

2 Scoop out 2 tablespoons of the mixture, and form it into a small patty. Repeat to form eight patties.

3 Heat 2 to 3 tablespoons of oil in a large pan over medium-low heat. Add the patties, working in batches if necessary, and cook until golden, 2 to 3 minutes per side. Transfer to a paper towel–lined plate.

4 Let cool completely before serving. The patties will seem soft at first but will firm up as they cool.

Storage

Store in an airtight container in the fridge for up to 3 days. To freeze, store in a freezer-safe airtight container for up to 2 months. To reheat, microwave for 20 to 30 seconds, adding 10-second intervals as needed, until warmed through. You can also place on a baking sheet and reheat in a 350°F (180°C) oven for 10 minutes, or until warmed through.

Tips

1. You may precook sweet potatoes in the oven (poke holes in the potatoes, and bake at 425°F/220°C for 45 to 50 minutes, until tender) or in the microwave (poke holes in the potatoes, and microwave for 5 to 6 minutes, until tender). Let cool, then peel and mash.

2. Tuna is high in mercury and is recommended to be avoided (or offered in moderation) for children under the age of two. Canned salmon is a good, lower-mercury alternative.

3. Egg-free? For this recipe, you may omit the egg completely! The patties will be slightly less moist on the inside but will still bind with the sweet potato. Place the patties in the fridge for 10 minutes to firm up before cooking.

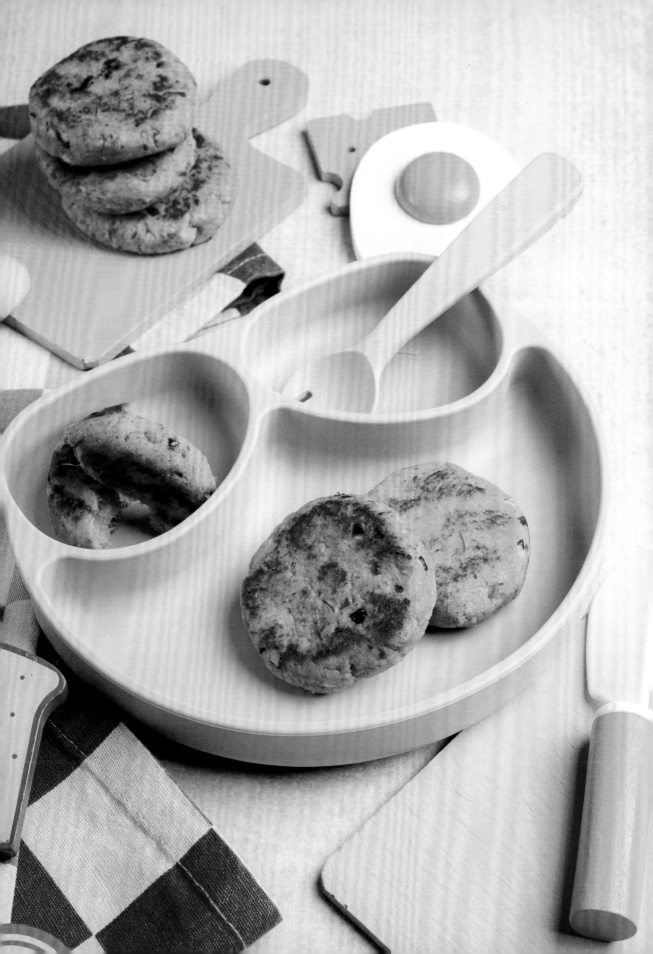

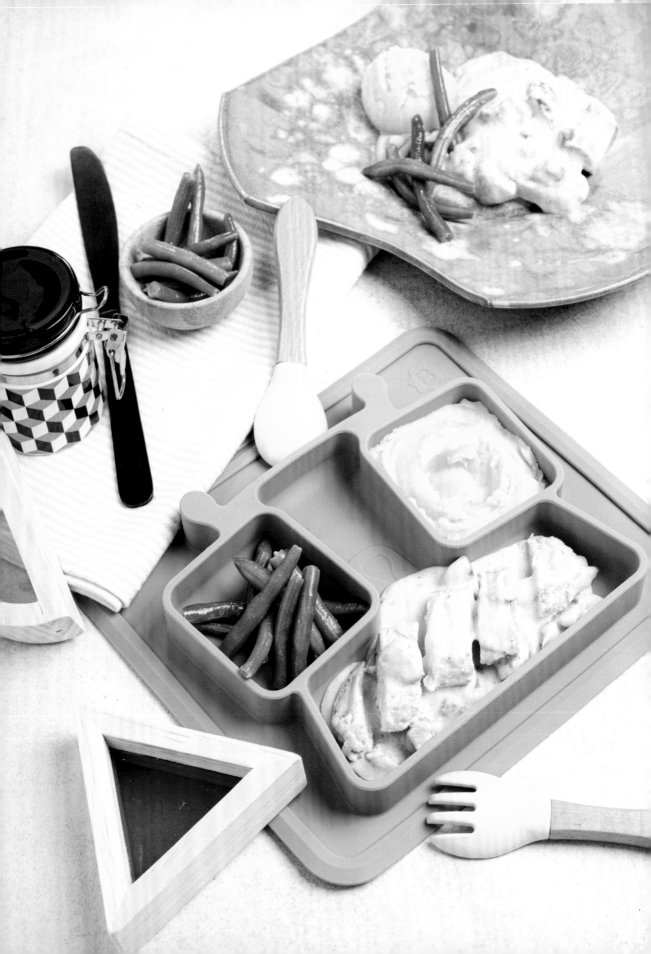

Creamy Mushroom Chicken

prep **15 minutes** / cook **20 minutes** / serves **2 adults & 2 children**

Sauce

½ cup (120 ml) half-and-half

¼ cup (60 ml) chicken stock

¼ cup (25 g) grated Parmesan

1½ teaspoons all-purpose flour

¼ teaspoon black pepper

Chicken

Four 4-ounce (113 g) thin-sliced chicken breasts (see Tip 1)

¼ teaspoon garlic powder

¼ teaspoon sweet paprika

2 tablespoons unsalted butter, divided

2 garlic cloves, minced

1¼ cups (114 g) sliced white mushrooms

Salt, to taste (optional)

Something about the combination of cream, mushrooms, and chicken is so warm and comforting. This creamy, mushroomy chicken dish is simple to make and packed with great flavor. I'll be honest: I'm not a big fan of the texture of mushrooms on their own, but I absolutely love the taste they add to this dish. Serve with potatoes and vegetables on the side.

1 Make the sauce: Whisk together the half-and-half, chicken stock, Parmesan, flour, and pepper in a small bowl, and set aside.

2 Season the chicken with garlic powder and paprika.

3 Melt 1 tablespoon of butter in a large frying pan over medium heat. Add the chicken, and cook until the center registers 165°F (75°C) on an instant-read thermometer, 4 to 5 minutes per side. Transfer the chicken to a plate, and set aside.

4 Melt the remaining 1 tablespoon of butter in the pan, and add the garlic, moving it around the pan until it begins to brown, 1 to 2 minutes.

5 Finely chop the mushrooms, and add them to the pan. Cook until tender, 3 to 5 minutes.

6 Reduce the heat to medium-low and pour the sauce into the pan. Cook until thickened, 3 to 5 minutes. Return the chicken to the pan, and add salt to taste (see Tips 2 and 3).

Storage

This creamy chicken is best served fresh but can be stored in an airtight container in the fridge for up to 3 days. Reheat the chicken and sauce in a large skillet over medium-low heat until warmed through, 2 to 3 minutes.

Tips

1. If you can't find thinly sliced chicken breasts, you can slice a chicken breast by placing your palm on top of the breast and carefully slicing the chicken in half horizontally, making two thin pieces.

2. If serving to a baby, slice the chicken into strips to make it easier to pick up and hold.

3. Remove baby's portion, and add salt to taste for the rest of the family.

One-Pot Chicken Pasta

prep **5 minutes** / cook **30 minutes** / serves **2 adults & 2 children**

1 pound (454 g) chicken breast (see Tip 1)

1 teaspoon garlic powder

½ teaspoon sweet paprika

1 tablespoon olive oil

½ cup (70 g) chopped yellow onion

1 teaspoon Italian seasoning

3 cups (720 ml) chicken broth

1½ cups (375 g) marinara sauce

1 cup (240 ml) heavy cream

8 ounces (227 g) penne (see Tip 2)

½ cup (57 g) shredded mozzarella

½ cup (50 g) grated Parmesan, plus more for serving

1 cup (60 g) fresh baby spinach, tightly packed

Salt, to taste (optional, see Tip 3)

It's so easy for the kitchen to become a mess when you're prepping dinner, but this no-fuss chicken pasta reduces the mess because it's all cooked in one pot. No need to cook the pasta separately because it cooks with the sauce. That means there's one fewer pot to clean, and you can get dinner on the table in no time!

1 Slice the chicken breast into 1-inch (2.5 cm) cubes, and season with garlic powder and paprika.

2 Heat the oil in a large pot over medium-high heat. Add the chicken in an even layer, and cook until no pink remains, about 3 minutes per side. Remove the chicken from the pot, and set aside.

3 To the same pot, add the onion and Italian seasoning. Cook, stirring occasionally, until the onion is softened, about 5 minutes.

4 Pour in the chicken broth, marinara sauce, and heavy cream, and stir. Bring the mixture to a boil, then stir in the penne.

5 Bring to a boil again, reduce the heat to medium-low, and simmer, stirring occasionally, until the pasta is al dente, 13 to 15 minutes.

6 Stir in the mozzarella, Parmesan, spinach, and cooked chicken, and simmer until the spinach is wilted and the cheese fully melts, 1 to 2 minutes. Add a splash of water if the sauce seems thick.

7 Top with a sprinkle of Parmesan, and serve.

Storage

Store in an airtight container in the fridge for up to 4 days. To reheat, microwave for 1 to 2 minutes, stirring halfway, until warmed through. You can also reheat in a large skillet over medium-low heat.

Tips

1. Feel free to swap the chicken with another protein or omit it altogether for a vegetarian option.

2. Penne pasta noodles are safe to serve whole to babies.

3. Remove baby's portion, and add salt to taste for the rest of the family.

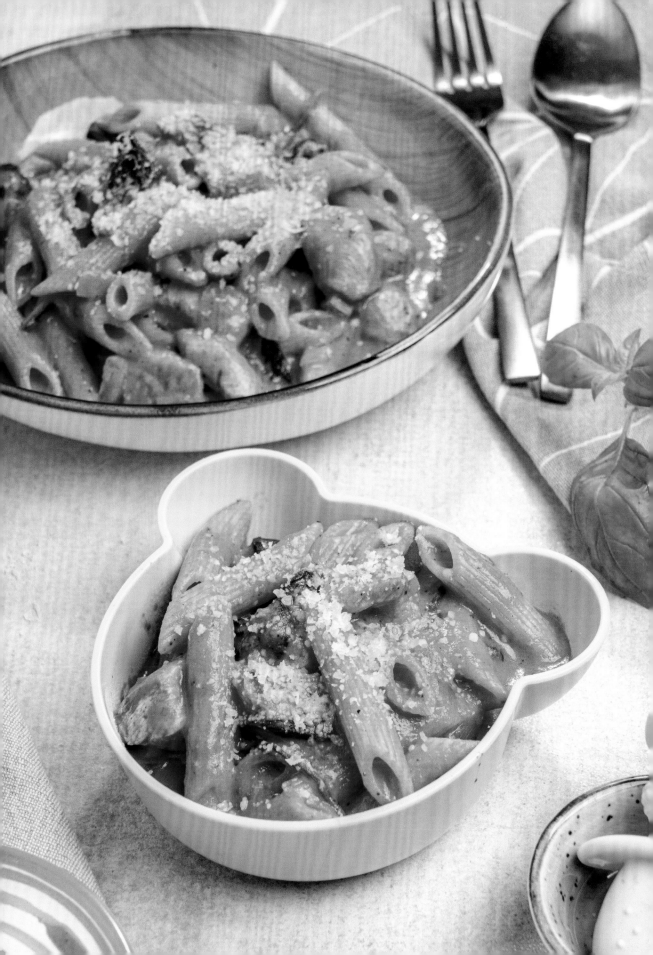

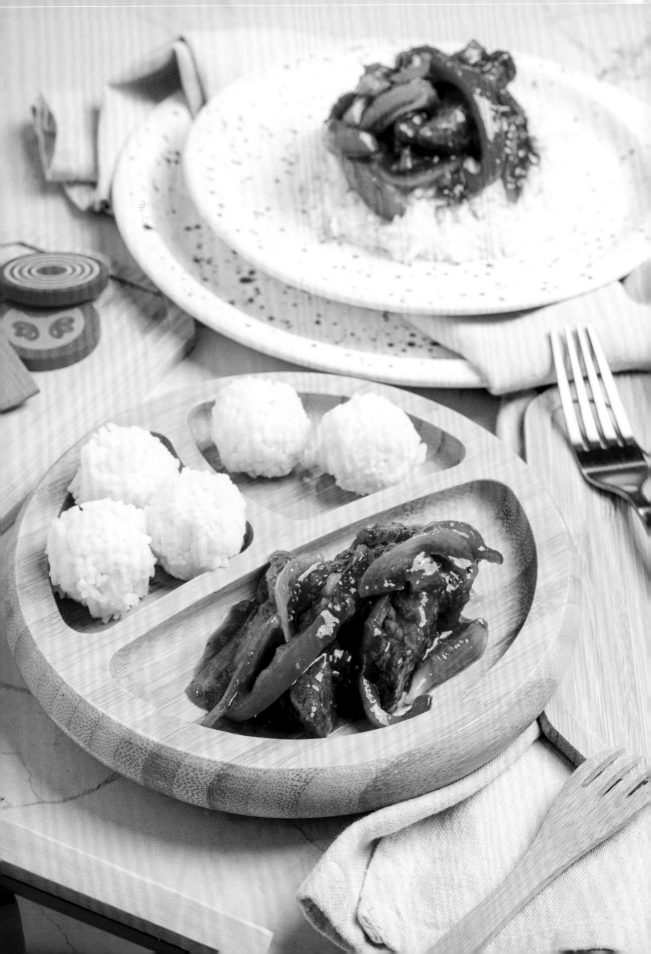

Beef Stir-Fry

prep **10 minutes** / cook **15 minutes** / serves **2 adults & 2 children**

Stir-Fry

1 pound (454 g) sirloin steak tips or flank steak, thinly sliced

Salt, to taste (optional)

Black pepper, to taste

2 tablespoons cornstarch

½ red bell pepper, ribs and seeds removed

½ green bell pepper, ribs and seeds removed

1 medium yellow onion

2 tablespoons olive oil, divided

Sauce

⅔ cup (160 ml) unsalted beef broth (see Tip 1)

¼ cup (60 ml) low-sodium soy sauce

2 tablespoons maple syrup

1 tablespoon cornstarch

1 teaspoon grated fresh ginger

½ teaspoon garlic powder

Skip the takeout, and make your own simple stir-fry at home! This meal comes together quickly and is as flavorful as can be. The sweet-and-savory sauce pairs so well with the tender beef and veggies for a meal you won't be able to resist! Serve this stir-fry over white rice (see Tip on page 155) or noodles.

1 Season the steak with salt (if using) and black pepper, and coat with cornstarch. Set aside to tenderize.

2 Slice the bell peppers and onion into strips, and set aside.

3 Heat 1 tablespoon of oil in a large frying pan over medium-high heat. Working in batches, add the steak and cook until browned on all sides, 3 to 4 minutes per side. Do not overcrowd the pan so the steak pieces sear properly. Transfer the steak to a plate, and set aside.

4 Add the remaining 1 tablespoon of oil to the pan. Add the peppers and onion, and sauté until tender-crisp, about 2 minutes. Transfer to the plate with the steak. Reduce the heat to medium.

5 Make the sauce: Whisk together the beef broth, soy sauce, maple syrup, cornstarch, ginger, and garlic powder in a small bowl until smooth, making sure no clumps remain. Pour the sauce into the pan, and whisk it until it thickens, 2 to 3 minutes.

6 Return the steak, peppers, and onion to the pan (see Tip 2). Simmer over low heat until everything is fully coated and cooked through, and serve (see Tip 3).

Storage

Store in an airtight container in the fridge for up to 3 days. To reheat, microwave for 1 to 2 minutes, until warmed through. You can also reheat in a large skillet over medium-low heat.

Tips

1. Swap the unsalted beef broth with unsalted chicken broth or water.

2. If preparing this for a baby, set aside a few pieces of steak and vegetables without adding them to the sauce.

3. A young baby may only gnaw on the steak without taking any actual bites, but even sucking on steak juices provides iron and nutrients! You can also shred the steak pieces into small bits to serve to baby.

DF EF NF GF

Pan-Seared Cajun Salmon

prep **5 minutes** / cook **10 minutes** / makes **3 filets**

1½ teaspoons sweet paprika

½ teaspoon salt (optional)

1 teaspoon garlic powder

½ teaspoon onion powder

½ teaspoon black pepper

½ teaspoon dried oregano

3 salmon fillets (about 6 ounces/170 g each, see Tip 1)

1 to 2 tablespoons olive oil

This is my go-to recipe for a classic salmon fillet that is moist and flaky and almost melts in your mouth with every bite! Pan-searing is my favorite method, but these fillets can be air-fried or oven-baked as well.

1 Mix the paprika, salt (if using), garlic powder, onion powder, pepper, and oregano in a small bowl. Sprinkle the mixture on all sides of the salmon fillets.

2 Heat the oil in a large skillet over medium heat. Add the salmon fillets, and cook undisturbed until the salmon is opaque two-thirds of the way up the sides, 3 to 4 minutes.

3 Flip the salmon, and cook until it is opaque and flaky when pulled apart with a fork, 1 to 2 minutes, depending on the thickness of the fillets (see Tip 2).

Storage

Store in an airtight container in the fridge for up to 3 days. To reheat, place on a baking sheet and bake in a 275°F (135°C) oven for 12 to 15 minutes, until warmed through.

Tips

1. Press the salmon fillets firmly to check for bones before using.

2. You may also bake this salmon in the oven at 400°F (200°C) for 12 to 15 minutes or air-fry at 390°F (200°C) for 8 to 10 minutes, until cooked through.

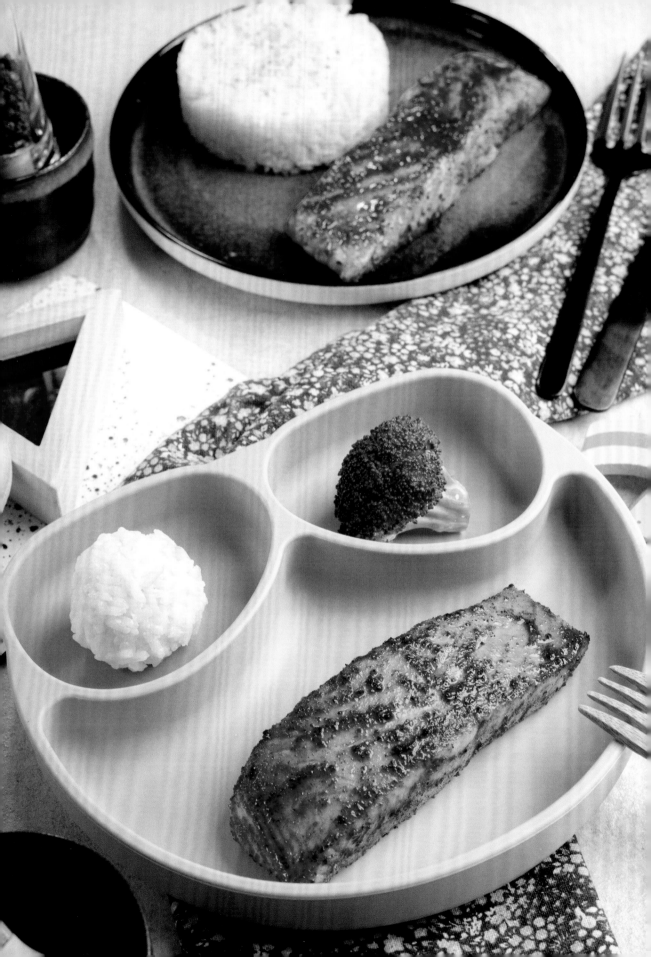

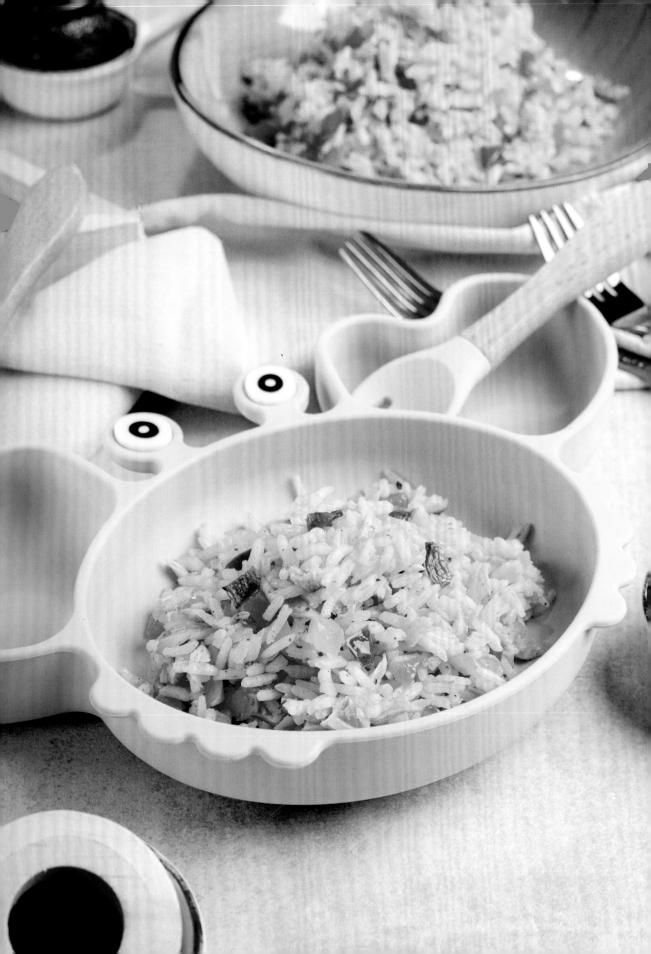

Salmon Rice

prep **10 minutes** / cook **5 minutes** / serves **2 adults & 2 children**

2 tablespoons olive oil

½ cup (70 g) finely chopped yellow onion

½ cup (70 g) finely chopped red and green bell peppers

½ teaspoon garlic powder

½ teaspoon sweet paprika

2 cooked salmon fillets (from Pan-Seared Cajun Salmon, page 152)

2 cups (400 g) cooked white rice

Salt, to taste (optional)

This salmon rice is a great way to both use up leftover white rice and elevate it! Everything comes together in minutes and can be enjoyed as a meal or as a side. Salmon is rich in fatty acids and omega-3s, making it a great source of healthy fats and protein to add to rice for a delicious, well-balanced meal.

1 Heat the oil in a medium pan over medium heat. Add the onion, bell peppers, garlic powder, and paprika, and sauté until the onion and bell peppers are soft and translucent, 3 to 5 minutes.

2 Remove from the heat, and set aside to cool. Be sure to keep all the juices from the sautéed veggies to add to the bowl with the remaining ingredients.

3 Shred the salmon with a fork.

4 Add the rice, salmon, and cooked veggies to a large bowl, and mix to combine. Season with salt to taste, and serve (see Tip).

Storage

Store in an airtight container the fridge for up to 3 days. To reheat, microwave for 2 minutes, or until warmed through.

Tip

· Rice can sometimes be difficult for babies to eat, so scoop out tablespoon-sized portions of the rice mixture and press firmly into small balls to make it easier for your little one to pick up and eat!

Creamy Avocado Pasta

prep **5 minutes** / cook **10 minutes** / serves **2 adults & 2 children**

- 8 ounces (227 g) spaghetti (or pasta of choice)
- 1 large ripe avocado, pitted
- 1 cup (60 g) baby spinach
- 1 garlic clove
- 1 tablespoon fresh lemon juice
- ¼ teaspoon salt (optional, see Tip 1)

Pasta doesn't get easier than this! It's rich, flavorful, and creamy without any dairy, and the bright green color makes it a fun meal for little ones. It takes no more than 15 minutes to whip up from start to finish and is perfect for a quick and easy weeknight dinner.

1 Bring a large pot of water to a boil, and cook the spaghetti according to the package directions. Drain, reserving ⅓ cup (80 ml) of the pasta water.

2 Scoop the avocado flesh into a high-powered blender. Add the spinach, garlic, lemon juice, pasta water, and salt (if using), and blend until smooth (see Tip 2). If the mixture is hard to blend, add 1 or 2 tablespoons of water.

3 Pour the sauce on top of the pasta, toss to coat, and serve (see Tip 3).

Storage

This sauce is best served fresh due to the natural oxidation of avocados, but any leftover sauce can be stored in an airtight container in the fridge for up to 2 days. You can eat this dish cold (like a pasta salad) or reheat it in the microwave for 20 to 30 seconds, until warmed through.

Tips

1. Remove baby's portion, and add salt to taste for the rest of the family.
2. Feel free to blend in some grated Parmesan for added flavor.
3. Pair with cooked, sliced chicken breast for some added protein.

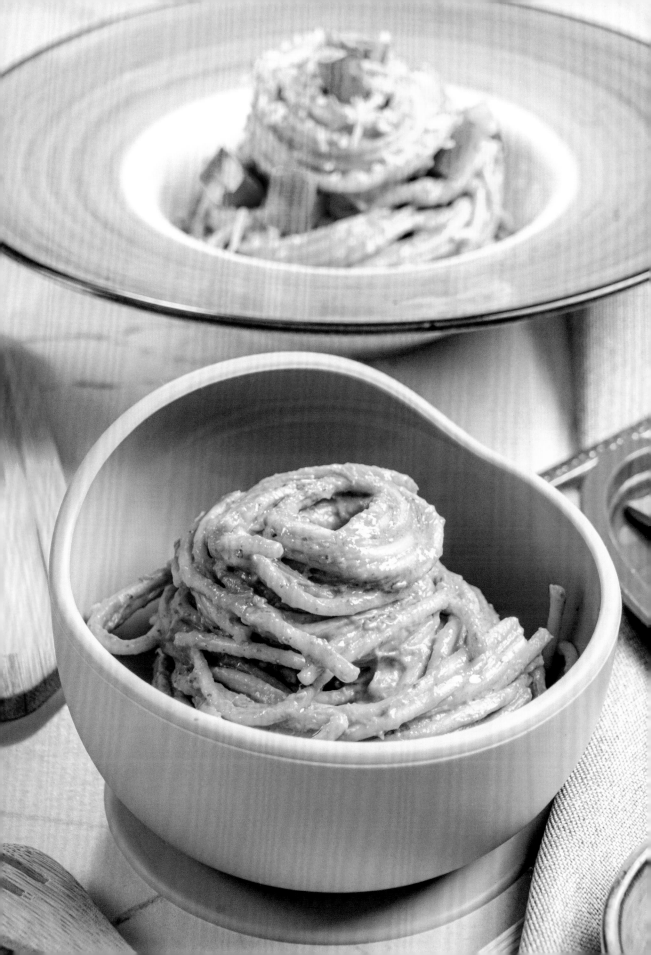

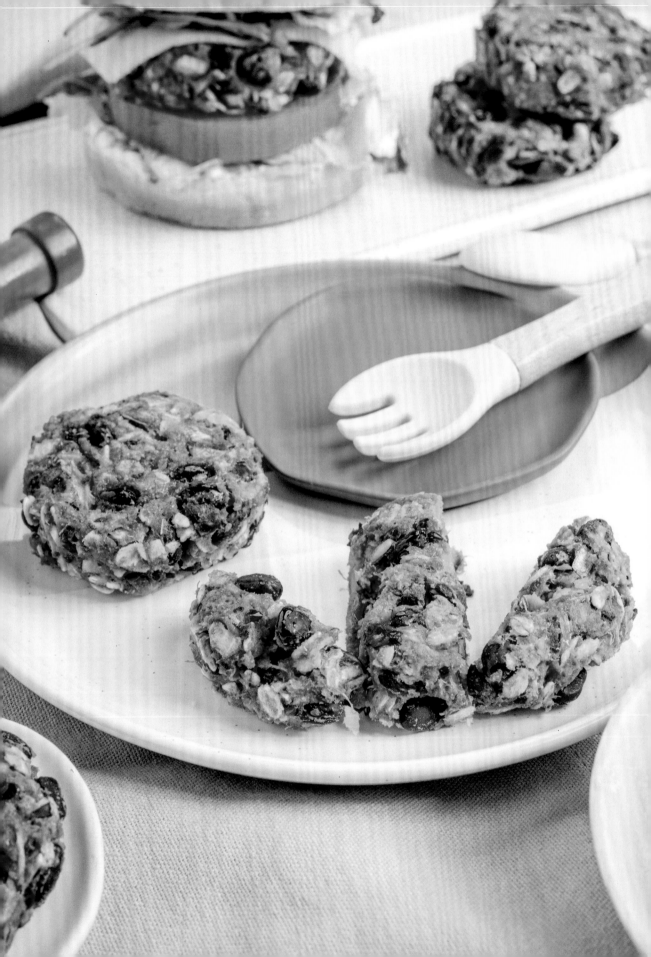

Black Bean & Sweet Potato Patties

prep **8 minutes** / cook **30 minutes** / makes **8 patties**

¾ cup (180 g) mashed cooked sweet potato (see Tip 1)

One 15-ounce (425 g) can black beans, drained and rinsed

⅓ cup (47 g) finely diced yellow onion

½ cup (45 g) old-fashioned rolled oats

1 teaspoon sweet paprika

1 teaspoon ground cumin

½ teaspoon garlic powder

½ teaspoon salt (optional)

These patties are a high-iron, nutrient-dense meal option that is so versatile! You can serve them in a bun, with a dip, or as is. The soft texture is perfect for babies, and the added spices are a great way to expand your little one's palette with a variety of flavors.

1 Preheat the oven to 375°F (190°C). Line a baking sheet with parchment paper.

2 Add the sweet potato and beans to a large bowl. Mash half of the beans with a fork, and leave the other half whole.

3 Add the onion, oats, paprika, cumin, garlic powder, and salt (if using), and mix to combine.

4 Use a ¼-cup (60 ml) measuring cup to scoop out equal portions of the mixture. Shape the portions, using damp hands to prevent the mixture from sticking, into ¾-inch-thick (2 cm) patties. Place the patties onto the baking sheet.

5 Bake for 30 minutes, or until firm to touch, flipping the patties halfway through to ensure even baking. Let cool completely before serving (see Tip 2).

Storage

Store in an airtight container in the fridge for up to 3 days. To freeze, store in a freezer-safe airtight container for up to 3 months. To reheat, microwave for 1 minute or heat in a large skillet over medium-low heat, until warmed through.

Tips

1. You may precook the sweet potato in the oven (poke holes in the potato, and bake at 425°F/220°C for 45 to 50 minutes, until tender) or in the microwave (poke holes in the potato, and microwave for 5 to 6 minutes, until tender). Let cool, then peel and mash.

2. If serving this to a baby, slice the patties into strips to make them easier to pick up and hold.

Veggie-Packed Beef Meatballs

prep **10 minutes** / cook **25 minutes** / makes **22 to 26 medium meatballs**

1 medium carrot, finely grated (about ¼ cup/ 55 g)

½ medium zucchini, finely grated (about ¼ cup/ 55 g)

1 pound (454 g) ground beef

¼ cup (24 g) panko breadcrumbs

¼ cup (25 g) grated Parmesan

1 egg (see Tip 1)

½ teaspoon Italian seasoning

½ teaspoon garlic powder

½ teaspoon onion powder

½ teaspoon salt (optional)

2 cups (500 g) marinara sauce

Spaghetti and meatballs are a classic, and these meatballs are tender, juicy, and never dry. I love adding in some grated veggies, which brings even more moisture to these flavorful and versatile meatballs. Serve them simmered in marinara sauce over pasta for a dinner the whole family will love!

1 Preheat the oven to 400°F (200°C). Line a baking sheet with parchment paper.

2 Use a cheesecloth, a clean kitchen towel, or your hands to squeeze all the moisture out of the carrot and zucchini. You should end up with about ¼ cup (55 g) of grated veggies.

3 Add the veggies, beef, panko breadcrumbs, Parmesan, egg, Italian seasoning, garlic powder, onion powder, and salt (if using) to a large bowl. Use your hands to mix all the ingredients together until just incorporated.

4 Scoop out tablespoon-sized portions of the mixture, and roll them into small balls.

5 Place the balls on the baking sheet, and bake for 20 minutes, flipping the meatballs halfway, until cooked through and no longer pink on the inside.

6 Simmer the marinara sauce in a large frying pan over medium heat. Add the meatballs, simmer for 5 minutes, and serve (see Tip 2).

Storage

Store in an airtight container in the refrigerator for up to 3 days. To freeze, arrange the meatballs in a single layer on a baking sheet, and freeze until solid. Transfer the meatballs to a freezer-safe bag with most of the air removed, and freeze for up to 2 months. To reheat, place on a baking sheet, cover with foil, and bake in a 300°F (150°C) oven for 15 minutes, or until warmed through.

Tips

1. Egg-free? Swap the egg with a flax egg (see page 55).
2. If serving this to a young baby, quarter the meatballs. You may also make jumbo-sized meatballs bigger than baby's fist.

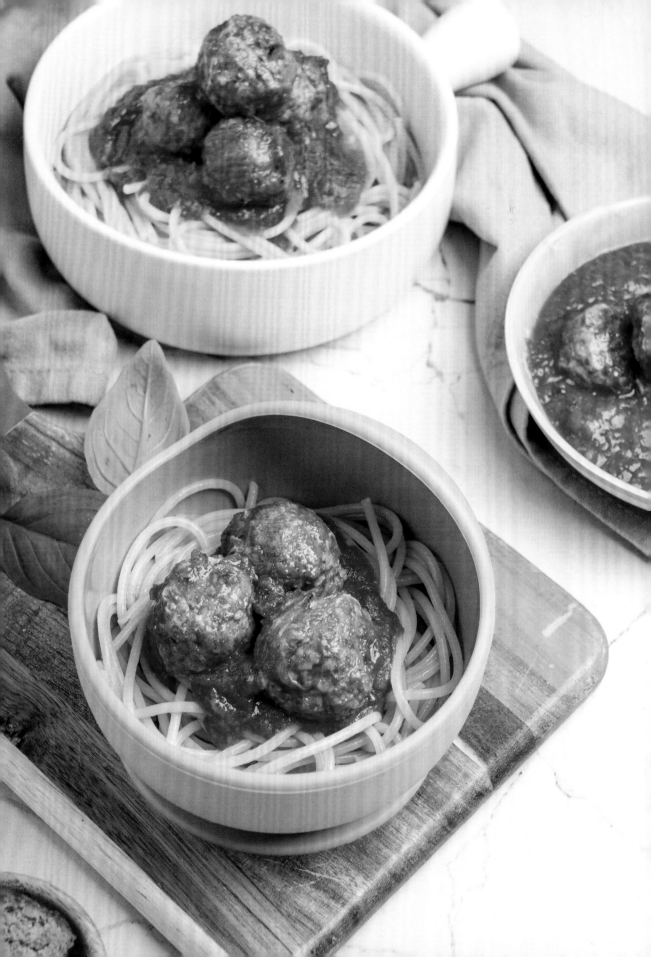

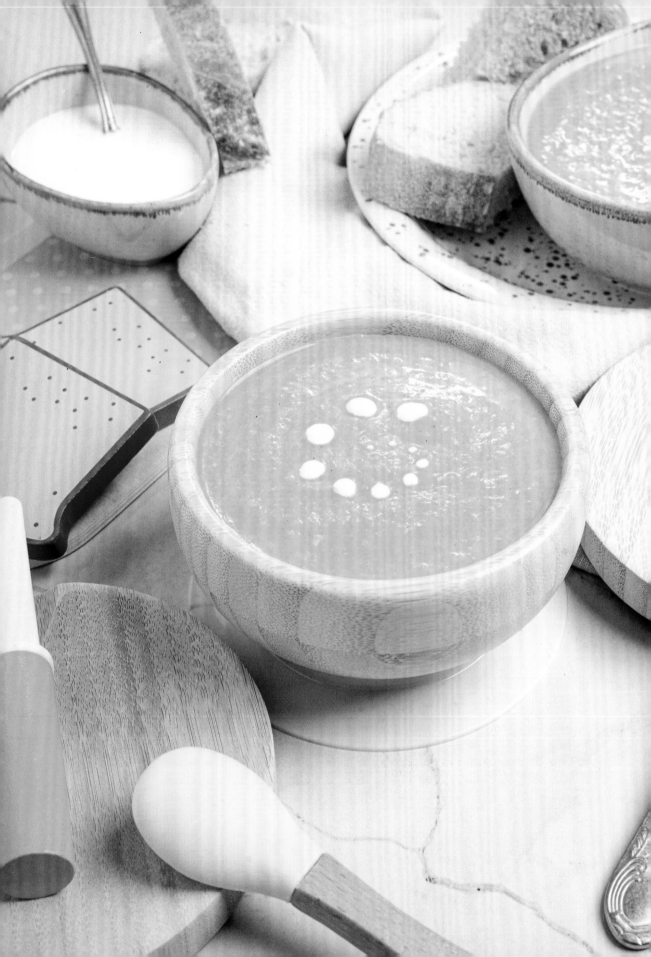

Creamy Pumpkin Soup

prep **5 minutes** / cook **30 minutes** / serves **2 adults & 2 children**

2 tablespoons unsalted butter

1 large yellow onion, finely diced

1 teaspoon pumpkin pie spice (see Tip 1)

¼ teaspoon garlic powder

2 cups (480 ml) chicken stock (see Tip 2)

One 15-ounce (425 g) can pumpkin puree

¼ cup (60 ml) heavy cream, plus more for serving (see Tip 3)

Salt, to taste (optional, see Tip 4)

If you're a pumpkin-all-year-round type of person, this creamy and comforting soup is calling your name. It's made with a can of pumpkin puree and just a few other ingredients, so it's a perfect weeknight dinner. I love using pumpkin puree for sweet treats, but this soup is a savory, fun twist. Serve it with a nice big loaf of bread for a filling meal.

1 Melt the butter in a large pot over medium heat. Add the onion and cook, stirring occasionally, until lightly browned and caramelized, about 10 minutes.

2 Add the pumpkin pie spice and garlic powder, and stir to combine. Stir in the chicken stock and pumpkin puree.

3 Reduce the heat to medium-low, and simmer until the soup thickens, 15 to 20 minutes. Add another splash of chicken stock if the puree is thick (see Tip 5).

4 Stir in the heavy cream and salt to taste (if using). Top with a drizzle of heavy cream, and serve.

Storage

Store in an airtight container in the fridge for up to 2 days. If you are planning to freeze leftovers, omit the heavy cream and stir it in after the soup is reheated to prevent curdling. Reheat the soup in a saucepan over medium-low heat, stirring occasionally, until warmed through.

Tips

1. No pumpkin spice? Replace it with 1 teaspoon ground cinnamon, ½ teaspoon ground nutmeg, and ½ teaspoon ground ginger.
2. Vegetarian? Swap the chicken stock with vegetable stock.
3. Dairy-free? Omit the heavy cream.
4. Remove baby's portion, and add salt to taste for the rest of the family.
5. If you prefer a smoother soup (without the bits of onions) you can blend it into a smooth puree before adding the cream.

Stuffed Shells Bake

prep **20 minutes** / cook **30 to 40 minutes** / makes **24 stuffed shells**

24 jumbo pasta shells
(see Tip 1)

2 tablespoons olive oil

1 small yellow onion,
finely diced

2½ cups (625 g) marinara
sauce

One 15-ounce (425 g)
container whole milk
ricotta

2½ cups (283 g) shredded
mozzarella, divided (see
Tip 2)

½ cup (50 g) grated
Parmesan

1 egg (see Tip 3)

1 teaspoon Italian
seasoning

This stuffed shells bake is one of my favorite meals to prep and assemble ahead of time. It's so easy to pop into the oven just before dinnertime to bake and serve. It freezes beautifully to store and serve at a later point and is a meal that you'll find yourself making again and again!

1 Preheat the oven to 375°F (190°C).

2 Bring a large pot of water to a boil, and cook the pasta shells according to package instructions. Drain the shells and rinse with cold water to stop the cooking and prevent the noodles from sticking. Let them sit in cold water until ready to use.

3 While the pasta cooks, prepare the sauce and cheese mixture. Heat the oil in a medium saucepan over medium heat. Add the onion, and cook until translucent, about 5 minutes.

4 Add the marinara sauce, and let it simmer and bubble for 5 minutes. Pour the sauce into the bottom of a 9 × 13-inch (23 × 33 cm) baking dish.

5 Mix the ricotta, 1½ cups (170 g) mozzarella, Parmesan, egg, and Italian seasoning in a large bowl until well combined. Scoop about 1 tablespoon of the cheese mixture into each shell, and place the stuffed shells in an even layer on top of the marinara sauce in the baking dish.

6 Sprinkle the remaining 1 cup (113 g) of mozzarella over the top of the shells.

7 Cover with foil, and bake for 20 minutes. Remove the foil, and bake for an additional 10 minutes, until the cheese fully melts. For golden, bubbly cheese, set the oven to high broil and broil for an additional 1 to 2 minutes, keeping a close eye on the cheese to ensure it doesn't burn.

Storage

Store in an airtight container in the fridge for up to 3 days. To reheat, microwave for 3 to 4 minutes or bake in a 300°F (150°C) oven for 15 to 20 minutes, until the shells are warmed through and the cheese is fully melted.

Tips

1. Boil a few extra jumbo pasta shells just in case some break while boiling.

2. Dairy-free? Replace the cheeses with dairy-free ricotta, dairy-free mozzarella, and dairy-free Parmesan (or nutritional yeast).

3. Egg-free? Swap the egg with 2 to 3 tablespoons of milk.

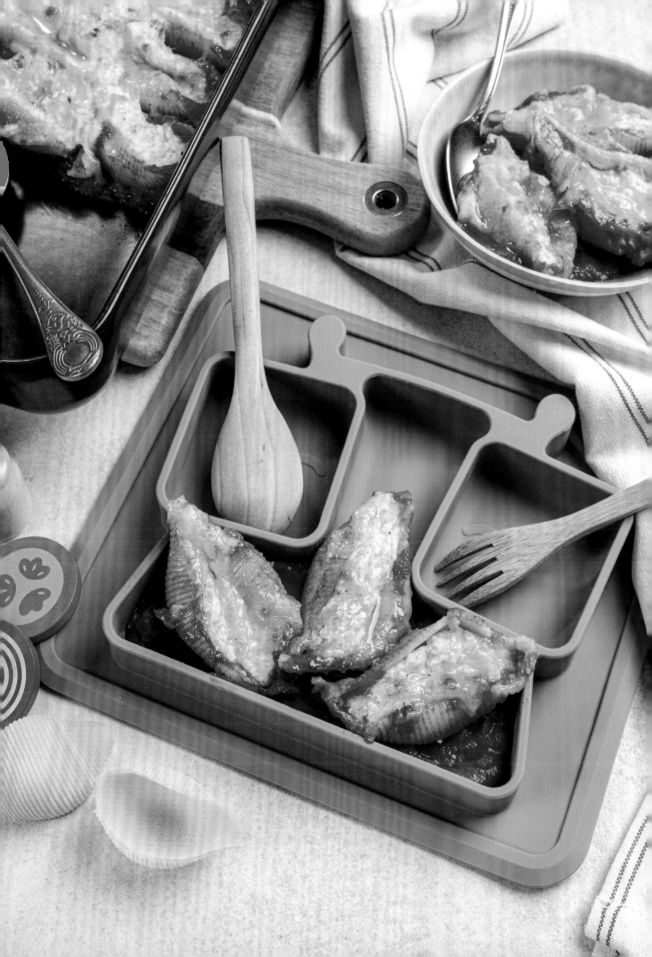

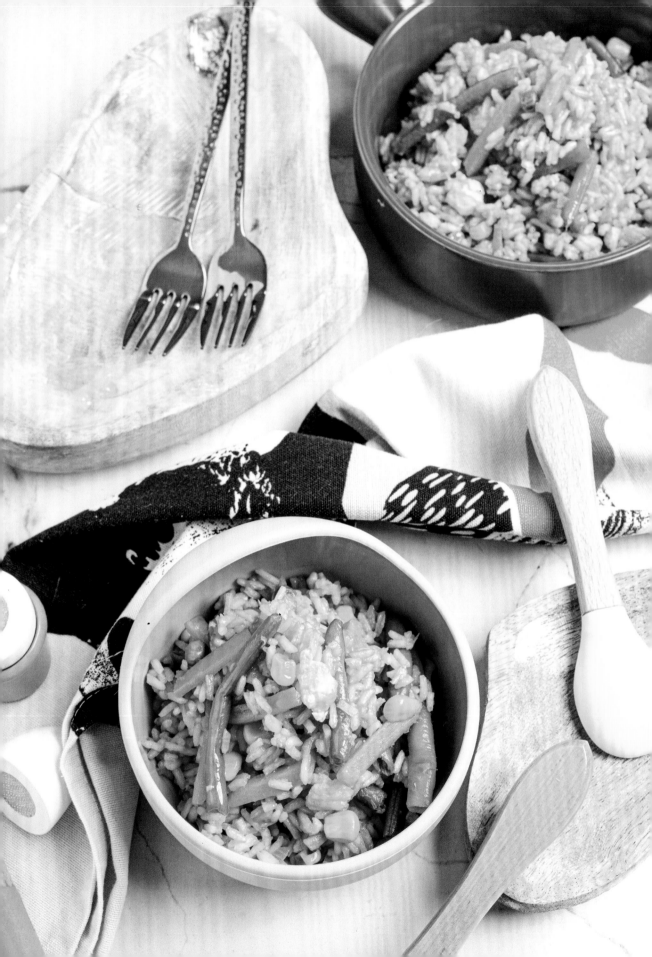

Vegetable Fried Rice

prep **10 minutes** / cook **10 minutes** / serves **3 adults & 3 children**

2 tablespoons olive oil, divided

3 eggs

1 medium yellow onion, diced

2 cups (240 g) frozen mixed vegetables

4 cups (800 g) cooled cooked white rice (see Tip 1)

3 tablespoons low-sodium soy sauce

2 tablespoons oyster sauce (optional)

Salt and black pepper, to taste (see Tip 2)

This fried rice is a great way to incorporate veggies and protein into an easy-to-make meal. Everything comes together in one pot and can be easily customized with your favorite add-ins. Serve it on its own or as a side for a quick dinner option!

1 Heat 1 tablespoon of oil in a large nonstick skillet or wok over medium heat.

2 Crack the eggs into a small bowl, whisk well, and add them to the pan, breaking them up into small pieces to cook, 2 to 3 minutes. Remove from the pan, and set aside.

3 Add the remaining 1 tablespoon of oil to the pan. Add the onion and frozen mixed vegetables to the pan, and cook until the onions are translucent and the veggies are warmed through, 5 minutes.

4 Add the rice, soy sauce, and oyster sauce (if using), and mix until all the rice grains are coated.

5 Return the scrambled eggs to the pan, season with salt and pepper (see Tip 2), and mix until well combined.

Storage

Store in an airtight container in the fridge for up to 3 days. To reheat, microwave for 1 to 2 minutes or heat in a skillet over medium-low heat, until warmed through.

Tips

1. Cold rice works best in this recipe, so use rice that is straight from the refrigerator.
2. Remove baby's portion, and add salt to taste for the rest of the family.
3. Feel free to add some chopped, cooked chicken breasts or thighs for an extra source of protein to make this chicken fried rice!

Parmesan-Crusted Salmon

prep **5 minutes** / cook **14 minutes** / makes **3 fillets**

3 salmon fillets (about 6 ounces/170 g each; see Tip 1)

Salt and black pepper, to taste (see Tip 2)

¼ cup (24 g) panko breadcrumbs

¼ cup (25 g) grated Parmesan

¼ teaspoon garlic powder

2 tablespoons unsalted butter, melted

Salmon is nutritious and rich in healthy fats that are crucial for baby and toddler development. This salmon has a crisp Parmesan coating on the outside and is moist and flaky on the inside. Pair it with your favorite sides for a dinner that's ready to serve in minutes!

1 Preheat the oven to 400°F (200°C). Line a baking sheet with parchment paper.

2 Season the salmon with salt and pepper, and place the fillets on the prepared baking sheet.

3 Mix the panko breadcrumbs, Parmesan, garlic powder, and melted butter in a small bowl to form a crumb coating.

4 Evenly distribute the coating on top of the salmon fillets, and press it in firmly so it sticks.

5 Bake for 12 to 14 minutes, depending on the thickness of the fillets, until the salmon is opaque and the crust is golden.

6 For a crispier, browned crust, set the oven to high broil, and broil for 1 minute.

Storage

Store in an airtight container in the fridge for up to 2 days. To reheat, place on a baking sheet and bake in a 275°F (135°C) oven for 12 to 15 minutes, until warmed through.

Tips

1. Press the salmon fillets firmly to check for bones before using.
2. Set aside a small piece of salmon without salt for baby, and season the remaining fillet pieces for the rest of the family.

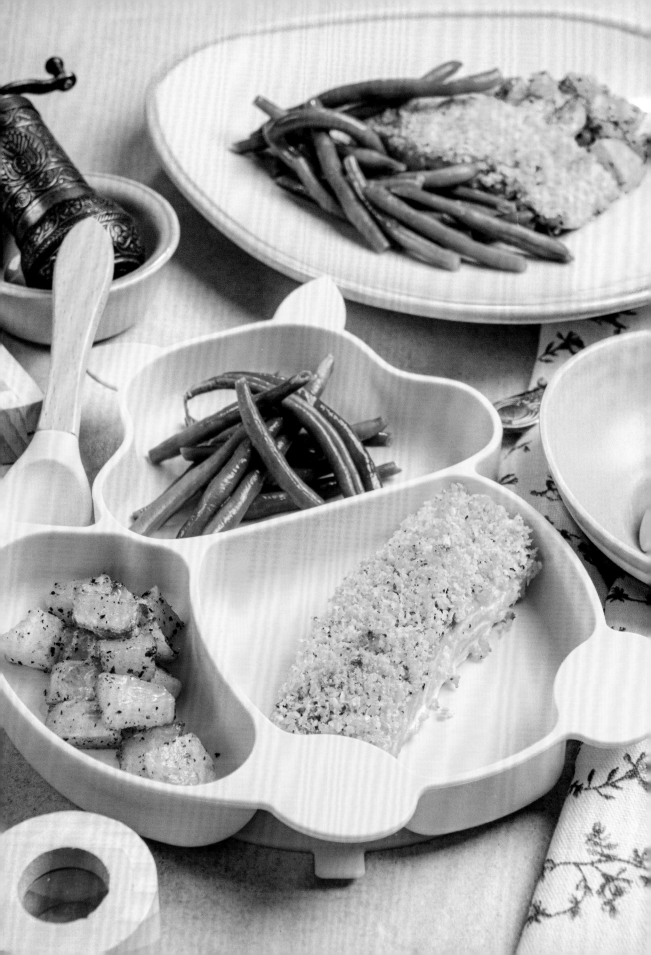

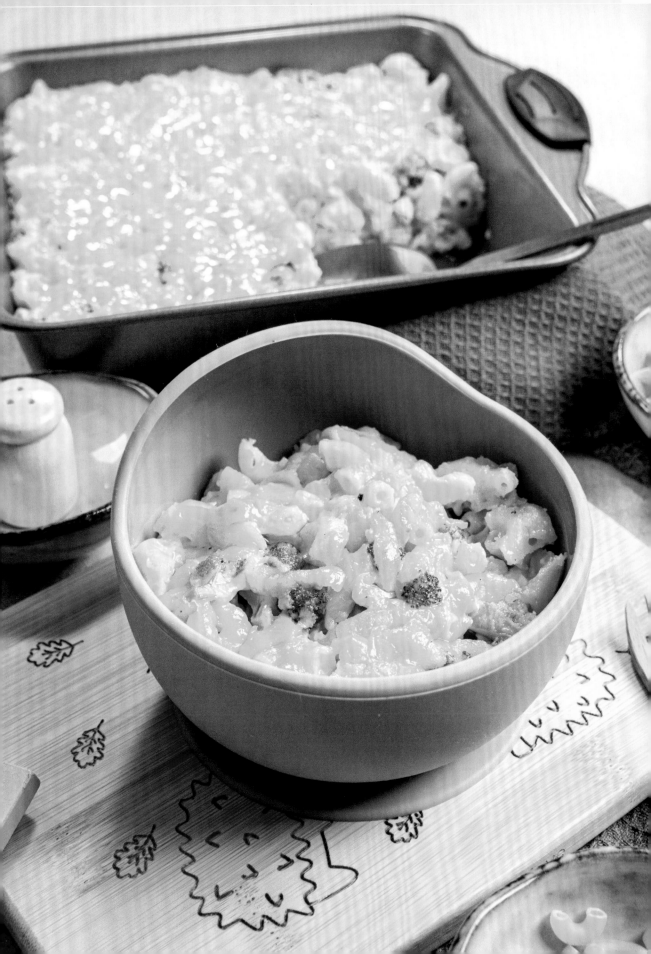

Broccoli Mac & Cheese Bake

prep **15 minutes** / cook **40 minutes** / serves **2 adults & 3 children**

Cooking spray (olive or avocado oil)

8 ounces (227 g) elbow macaroni

3 tablespoons unsalted butter

2 tablespoons all-purpose flour

1½ cups (360 ml) whole milk

½ cup (120 ml) heavy cream

2½ cups (285 g) shredded sharp cheddar, divided

½ teaspoon salt (optional)

⅛ teaspoon black pepper

2 cups (180 g) broccoli florets (see Tip 1)

I'm a firm believer in the magic that happens when veggies meet cheese, and this macaroni and cheese bake is a testament to that magic. The creamy cheese sauce and pasta come together on the stove and finish in the oven for a cheesy, tender bake. The broccoli adds the perfect texture and taste and is a great way to incorporate some veggies into this classic dish.

1 Preheat the oven to 350°F (180°C). Spray an 8-inch (20 cm) square baking pan with cooking spray.

2 Bring a large pot of water to a boil, and cook the macaroni according to the package directions but for 1 minute less than al dente. Drain and set aside.

3 Melt the butter in a large saucepan over medium heat. Stir in the flour, and continuously whisk until smooth and golden in color, about 1 minute.

4 Slowly add the milk and heavy cream, and mix until smooth, about 3 minutes.

5 Add 2 cups (228 g) of cheddar, and whisk until it fully melts and the sauce is smooth and thick, 3 to 5 minutes. Season with salt (if using) and pepper.

6 Add the broccoli florets to a medium microwave-safe bowl with 1 tablespoon of water, cover with a plate, and microwave for 3 minutes. Drain the liquid, and use kitchen scissors to cut the broccoli into small pieces.

7 Add the pasta and broccoli to the cheese sauce, and mix until fully incorporated. Pour the pasta mixture into the baking pan, and sprinkle the remaining ½ cup (57 g) of cheese on top.

8 Bake for 25 to 30 minutes, until golden brown (see Tip 2). Serve.

Storage

Store in an airtight container or covered in the baking dish in the fridge for up to 3 days or in the freezer for up to 3 months. To reheat, thaw at room temperature for 20 to 25 minutes and then bake in a 300°F (150°C) oven for 30 to 35 minutes, until warmed through. You also can microwave portions for 2 to 3 minutes, until warmed through.

Tips

1. Feel free to add some other steamed veggies like carrots into the mix!

2. No time to bake? You can enjoy this pasta straight from the stovetop. Let it simmer for an additional 2 to 3 minutes before serving. It will be looser in texture but still fully cooked and delicious!

(DF) (EF) (NF)

Sheet Pan Chicken Fajitas

prep **10 minutes** / cook **25 minutes** / serves **2 adults & 2 children**

Fajita Seasoning
1 tablespoon chili powder
1 teaspoon sweet paprika
1 teaspoon salt (optional, see Tip 1)
½ teaspoon onion powder
¼ teaspoon ground cumin
¼ teaspoon black pepper
¼ teaspoon garlic powder

Fajitas
1 pound (454 g) chicken breast or boneless chicken thighs
3 small bell peppers (mixed colors), ribs and seeds removed
1 large yellow onion
2 tablespoons olive oil
½ lime
Eight 8-inch (20 cm) flour tortillas, for serving

Toppings (optional)
Sour cream
Shredded cheddar
Avocado slices

Sheet pan meals are a lifesaver when it comes to making dinner for the whole family. Just pop everything onto a tray, bake, and serve! These chicken fajitas bake quickly and can be customized with your favorite sides and toppings for a meal everyone in the family will love.

1 Preheat the oven to 400°F (200°C).

2 Make the fajita seasoning: Mix the chili powder, paprika, salt (if using), onion powder, cumin, black pepper, and garlic powder in a small bowl.

3 Slice the chicken into thin strips. Thinly slice the bell peppers and onion (see Tip 2).

4 Place the chicken, peppers, and onion on a large baking sheet. Drizzle the oil and fajita seasoning over the top, and mix to coat.

5 Bake for 20 to 25 minutes, stirring halfway through, until the vegetables are tender and the chicken is cooked through.

6 Remove from the oven, and squeeze lime juice over the fajitas.

7 Serve with warm tortillas, and top with sour cream, shredded cheddar, and avocado slices (if using).

Storage
Store in an airtight container in the fridge for up to 3 days. Reheat in the microwave for 1 or 2 minutes or heat in a large skillet over medium-low heat, until warmed through.

Tips
1. If preparing this for a baby, eliminate the salt from the seasoning mixture. Remove baby's portion, and add salt to taste for the rest of the family.
2. Thin strips are easier for beginner eaters to pick up and hold, but feel free to dice the chicken and veggies into smaller pieces if your little one has developed the pincer grasp.

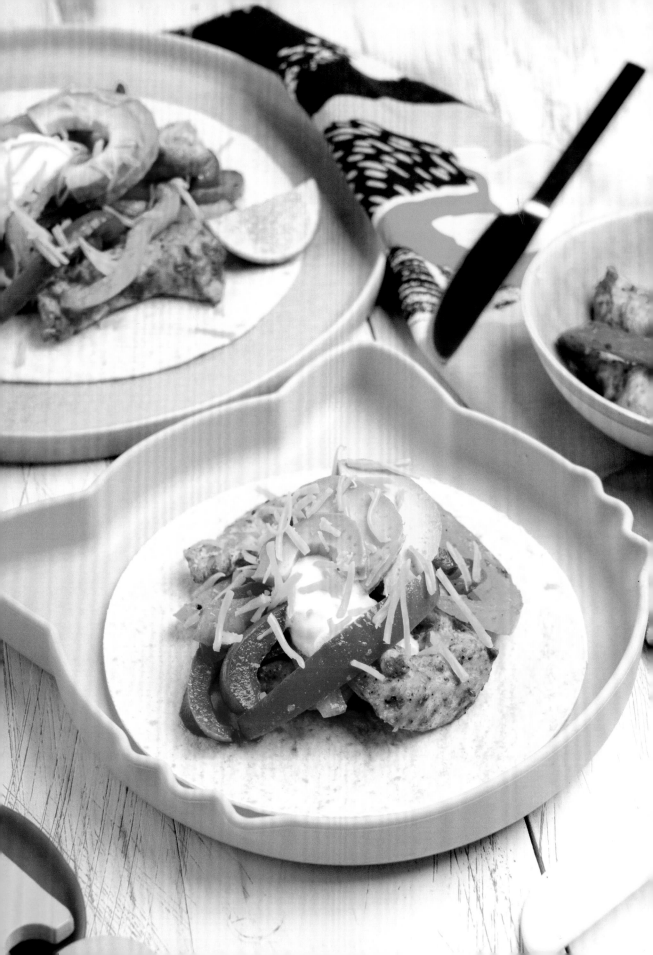

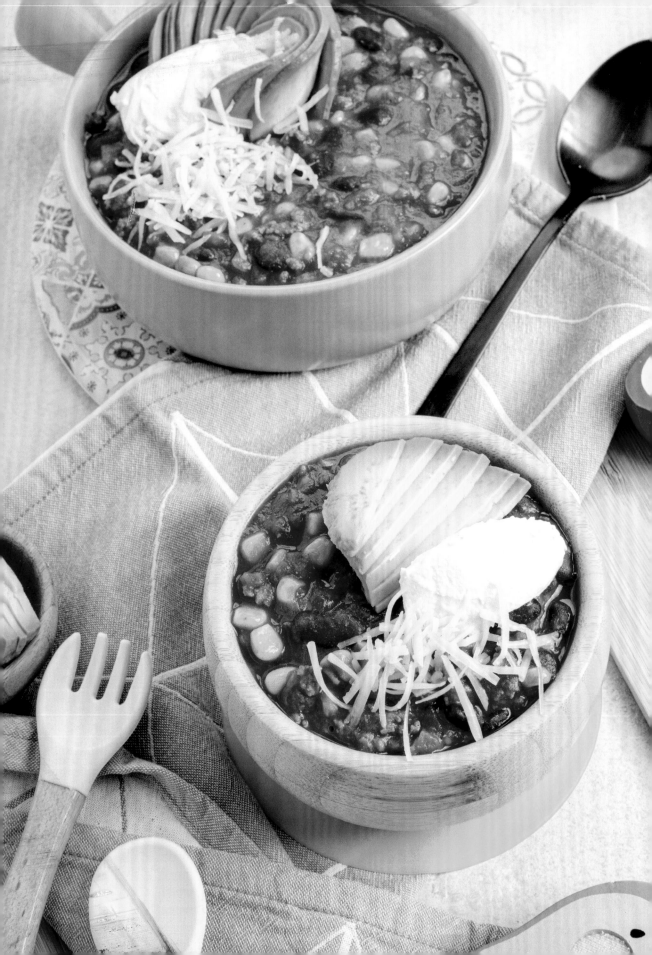

Taco Chili

prep **10 minutes** / cook **30 minutes** / serves **4 adults & 2 children**

Taco Seasoning (see Tip 1)
1 tablespoon chili powder
1 teaspoon ground cumin
1 teaspoon sweet paprika
1 teaspoon black pepper
1 teaspoon salt (optional)
¼ teaspoon garlic
   powder
¼ teaspoon onion
   powder
¼ teaspoon dried
   oregano

Taco Chili
1 pound (454 g) ground
   beef
1 cup (140 g) finely
   chopped yellow onion
One 15-ounce (425 g) can
   black beans, drained
   and rinsed
One 15-ounce (425 g) can
   red kidney beans,
   drained and rinsed
One 15-ounce (425 g) can
   corn kernels, drained
   and rinsed
One 15-ounce (425 g) can
   diced tomatoes
1 cup (240 ml) tomato
   sauce
Salt and black pepper,
   to taste (see Tip 2)

Toppings (optional)
Sour cream
Shredded cheddar
Avocado slices

This taco chili is a warm, comforting meal that comes together in one pot. It is packed with protein and iron from the beef and beans and reheats perfectly for leftovers the next day. Dump all the ingredients into a pot to cook, and you've got a simple meal for the whole family! It can be served as is or over rice.

1 Make the taco seasoning: Mix the chili powder, cumin, paprika, pepper, salt (if using), garlic powder, onion powder, and oregano in a small bowl.

2 Add the beef to a large pot over medium heat, and break it up. When it begins to brown, add the taco seasoning and onion, and cook until the beef is fully browned and no pink remains, 8 to 10 minutes.

3 Add the black beans, kidney beans, corn, diced tomatoes, and tomato sauce to the pot, and stir well. Reduce the heat to medium-low, and cook until thickened, about 20 minutes.

4 Add salt and pepper, and serve with sour cream, cheddar, and avocado slices (if using) on top.

Storage
Store in an airtight container in the fridge for up to 3 days or in the freezer for up to 6 months. Thaw frozen chili overnight in the fridge. Reheat in a pot over medium heat, stirring occasionally, until warmed through.

Tips
1. You can use a 1-ounce (28 g) packet of taco seasoning instead of making your own.
2. If serving to a baby, remove baby's portion from the pot, and add salt to taste for the rest of the family.

Garlic Butter Chicken Breast

prep **10 minutes** / cook **10 minutes** / makes **4 chicken breasts**

¼ cup (33 g) all-purpose flour

½ teaspoon sweet paprika

½ teaspoon garlic powder

½ teaspoon onion powder

½ teaspoon salt (optional)

Four 4-ounce (113 g) thin-sliced chicken breasts, at room temperature (see Tips 1 and 2)

2 tablespoons olive oil

3 garlic cloves, minced

½ cup (120 ml) chicken stock

4 tablespoons unsalted butter

1 teaspoon dried parsley or 1 tablespoon chopped fresh parsley

Black pepper, to taste

I love a good meal that can be prepped in one pan, and this garlic butter chicken definitely hits the spot. The chicken comes out moist and tender, and the garlic butter sauce adds extra juiciness that you won't be able to resist!

1 Whisk together the flour, paprika, garlic powder, onion powder, and salt (if using) in a shallow bowl. Dredge the chicken in the mixture, shaking off any excess flour.

2 Heat the oil in a large pan over medium-high heat. Add the chicken, and cook until golden brown, 4 to 5 minutes on one side and 3 to 4 minutes on the other. You may need to cook the chicken in batches. Transfer to a plate to rest.

3 Reduce the heat to medium, and add the garlic. Cook until it begins to brown slightly, about 1 minute, moving it around the pan and watching closely so it doesn't burn.

4 Add the chicken stock, and stir, scraping the pan. Add the butter, and stir it until it melts. Stir in the parsley.

5 Return the chicken to the pan, and season with salt and pepper (see Tip 3). Baste the chicken in the garlic butter sauce, simmer for 1 minute, and serve (see Tip 4).

Storage

Store in an airtight container in the fridge for up to 3 days. To reheat, place a small amount of water in a large skillet (enough to cover the bottom of the pan), and heat over medium heat. Add the chicken to the skillet, cover, and cook for about 5 minutes, or until the chicken is warmed through. This helps prevent the chicken from drying out.

Tips

1. Be sure the chicken is at room temperature before seasoning to help it cook more evenly.
2. If you can't find thinly sliced chicken breasts, you can slice a chicken breast by placing your palm on top of the breast and carefully slicing the chicken in half horizontally, making two thin pieces.
3. Remove baby's chicken from the pan, and add salt to taste for the rest of the family.
4. Slice the chicken in strips if serving to a young baby, or dice into small pieces if serving to a baby who has developed the pincer grasp.

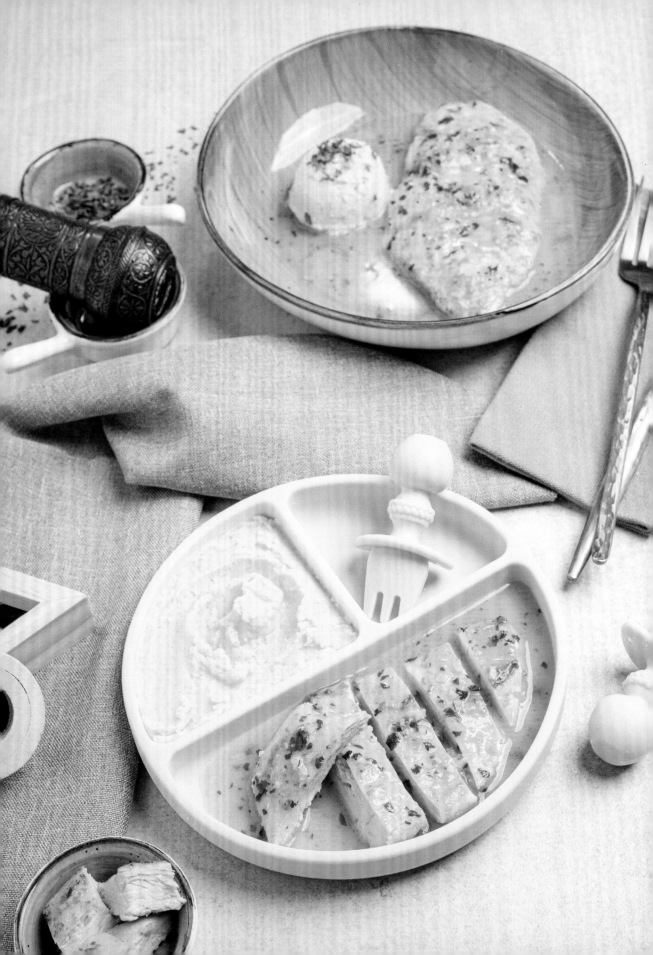

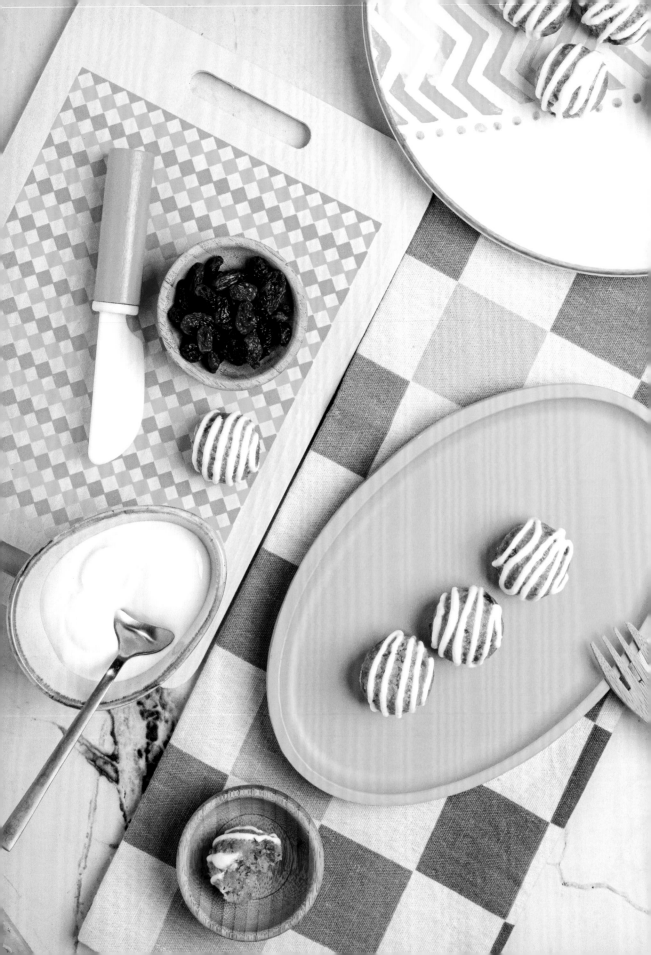

Snacks & Treats

Something about the word "snack" seems to make everything more appealing. Once my boys hear the word, they're immediately attentive. All of a sudden, they have the best appetites—even if they barely ate the meal that was offered just a few minutes before. I love to make the best of snack time and provide nutritious snacks that are still filling and tasty. The snacks and treats in this chapter are made with simple ingredients, are quick to prepare, and taste delicious. You may have to stop yourself from snacking on the whole batch before your little one gets a bite!

Banana Cookie Bars

prep **5 minutes** / cook **30 minutes** / makes **8 bars**

½ cup (125 g) mashed overripe banana (from about 1 large banana)

2 tablespoons natural peanut butter

3 tablespoons milk

½ cup (50 g) almond flour

½ cup (50 g) oat flour

¼ teaspoon ground cinnamon

½ teaspoon baking powder

¼ cup (43 g) chocolate chips, divided (optional, see Tip)

These banana cookie bars are packed with nutrients and healthy fats. They are naturally sweetened with bananas, and all the ingredients come together in one bowl. Add some chocolate chips for a decadent, soft, and chewy treat.

1 Preheat the oven to 350°F (180°C). Line a 9 × 5-inch (23 × 13 cm) loaf pan with parchment paper.

2 Whisk together the mashed banana, peanut butter, and milk in a large bowl until smooth.

3 Add the almond flour, oat flour, cinnamon, and baking powder, and mix until combined.

4 Fold in about 3 tablespoons of chocolate chips (if using), pour the mixture into the loaf pan, and spread into an even layer. Sprinkle the remaining chocolate chips on top.

5 Bake for 30 minutes, or until the edges are golden brown and the top is firm to touch.

6 Let cool completely, and slice into eight squares.

Storage

Store in an airtight container at room temperature for up to 2 days or in the fridge for up to 4 days. To freeze, store in a freezer-safe airtight container for up to 3 months. Reheat in the microwave for 20 to 30 seconds, until warmed through.

Tip

· The chocolate chips add a touch of added sweetness but can be omitted if serving to a baby.

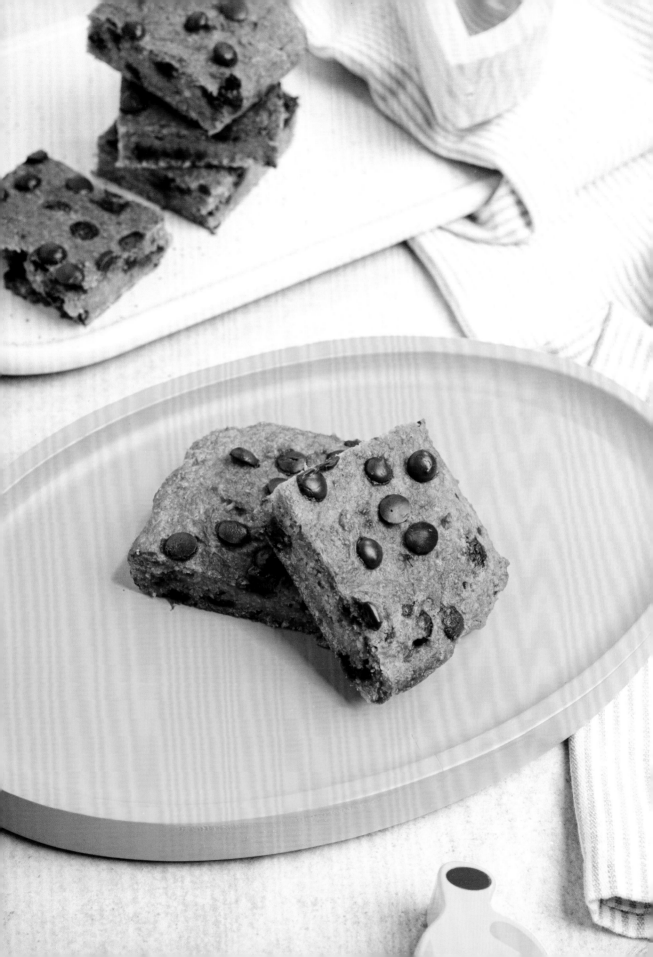

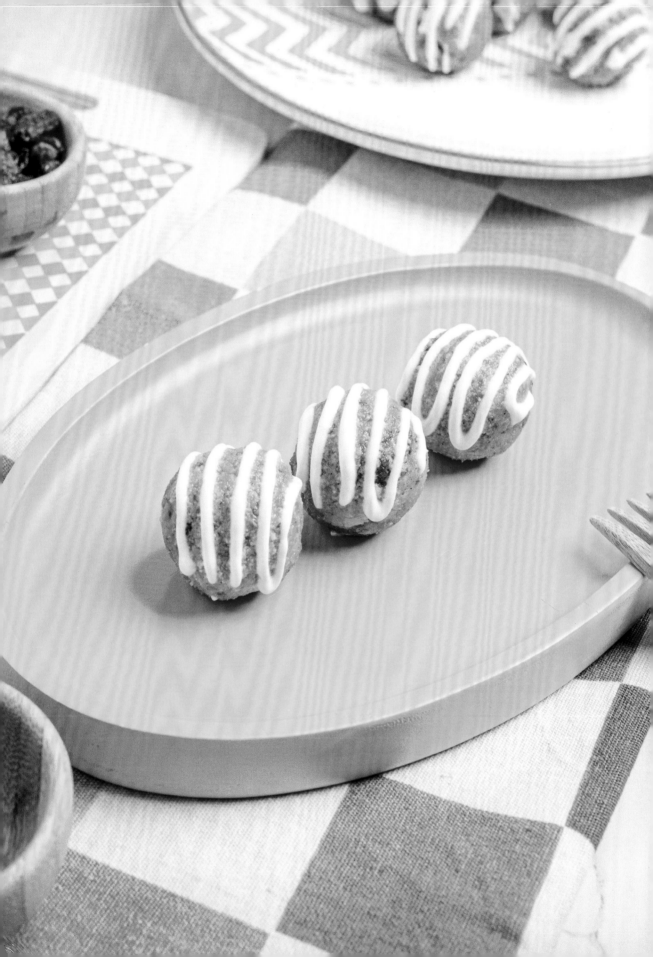

No-Bake Carrot Cake Bites

prep **5 minutes** / makes **10 to 12 balls**

⅔ cup (147 g) packed finely grated carrots

⅓ cup (67 g) raisins

1 cup (100 g) almond flour

½ teaspoon ground cinnamon

½ teaspoon ground ginger

¼ teaspoon ground nutmeg

Plain unsweetened yogurt (optional)

Desiccated coconut (optional)

If you love the taste of carrot cake but don't have the time (or energy!) to make one from scratch, you're going to love these soft, spiced, no-bake carrot cake bites. Add a few ingredients to a food processor, pulse into a smooth mixture, and roll into balls. They are naturally sweetened with raisins, and I promise they will become a go-to treat for the whole family!

1 Add the carrots, raisins, almond flour, cinnamon, ginger, and nutmeg to a food processor (not a blender; see Tip 1) and pulse on the puree setting until combined into a moist dough. Scrape down the sides of the food processor as needed for even pulsing.

2 Scoop out tablespoon-sized portions of the batter, and roll them into small balls.

3 Place the balls on a plate, and set in the fridge for 10 minutes to firm before serving.

4 Drizzle some yogurt (if using) on top or roll them in coconut (if using) for a fun touch (see Tips 2 and 3).

Storage

Store in an airtight container in the fridge for up to 2 days. To freeze, store in a freezer-safe airtight container for up to 1 month. Thaw at room temperature before serving.

Tips

1. It's important to use a food processor for this recipe because a blender will not be powerful enough to break down the mixture without added moisture.
2. If serving to a young baby, quarter the cake bites.
3. If you are planning on freezing any leftover cake bites, do not top them with yogurt.

Raspberry Peach Frozen Yogurt Bark

prep **8 minutes** / chill **2 hours** / makes **16 pieces**

½ cup (75 g) raspberries

One 15-ounce (425 g) can unsweetened sliced peaches, drained, divided

2 cups (480 g) plain whole milk Greek yogurt

2 tablespoons maple syrup (optional)

Toppings

¼ cup (38 g) raspberries, sliced

¼ cup (25 g) finely crushed granola

This frozen yogurt bark is a less-messy way of enjoying yogurt with all of your favorite toppings. It is so creamy from the Greek yogurt with bursts of sweetness from the raspberries and peaches. Top it with all of your favorite toppings for a nutritious snack. Offer it to little ones who are teething for some great gum relief!

1 Line a baking sheet with parchment paper.

2 In a blender, blend the raspberries and half of the peaches into a puree.

3 Transfer to a bowl with the yogurt and maple syrup (if using), and mix to combine.

4 Pour the mixture into the baking pan, and spread it in a smooth, even layer.

5 Slice the remaining peaches into thin strips, and spread them and the sliced raspberries evenly across the top. Sprinkle the granola over both.

6 Place the pan in the freezer for at least 2 hours to harden.

7 Break the bark into small pieces (see Tip). Let sit at room temperature to soften slightly before serving.

Storage

To freeze, store in a freezer-safe bag with most of the air removed for up to 3 months.

Tip

- Break the bark into mini, bite-sized pieces for a baby so that they are easier to eat.

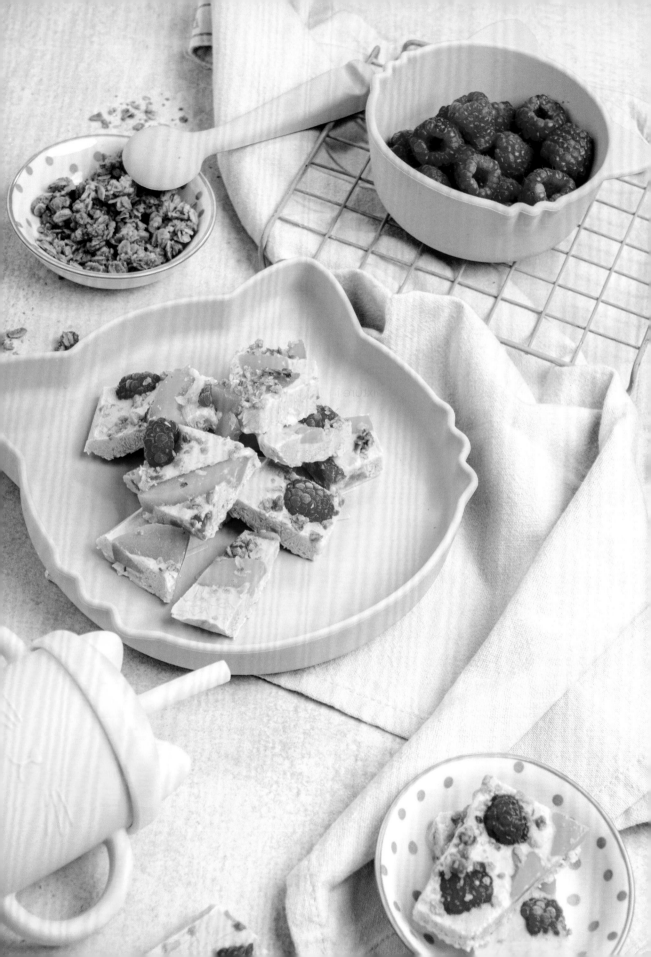

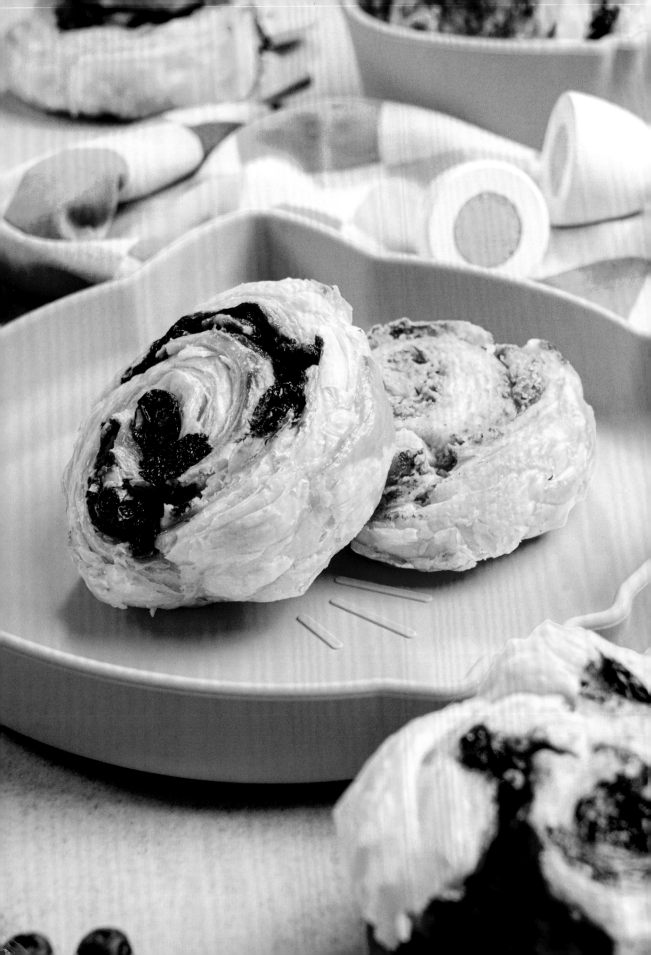

Blueberry Cheesecake Pinwheels

All-purpose flour, for dusting

1 sheet (245 g) puff pastry, thawed

1 teaspoon maple syrup (optional)

3 ounces (85 g) cream cheese, softened (see Tip 1)

1 cup (150 g) blueberries, roughly chopped

1 egg (see Tip 2)

Powdered sugar, for dusting (see Tip 3)

Peanut Butter Banana Pinwheels

All-purpose flour, for dusting

1 sheet (245 g) puff pastry, thawed

¼ cup (63 g) natural peanut butter

1 large banana, sliced

1 teaspoon ground cinnamon

Powdered sugar, for dusting (see Tip 3)

1 egg (see Tip 2)

Storage

Store in an airtight container in the refrigerator for up to 3 days. To freeze, store in a freezer-safe bag for up to 1 month. Reheat in a 350°F (180°C) oven for 10 minutes, or until warmed through.

Tips

1. Swap the cream cheese with mascarpone cheese for a lower-sodium option.

2. To make these pinwheels egg-free, swap the egg with melted butter or melted coconut oil to brush on top of the pieces before baking.

3. Serve to baby as is, and dust some powdered sugar on top for everyone else!

Flaky Fruity Pinwheels

prep **10 minutes** / cook **25 minutes** / makes **8 pinwheels**

These pinwheels are so easy to make with only a few ingredients and are the perfect sweet treat. They are flaky in texture and melt in the mouth—it'll be hard to eat just one! Each bite is bursting with sweetness that you won't be able to resist.

Blueberry Cheesecake Pinwheels

1 Preheat the oven to 400°F (200°C). Line a baking sheet with parchment paper.

2 Dust a work surface with flour and then unfold the puff pastry sheet onto the surface.

3 Mix the maple syrup (if using) and cream cheese in a small bowl until smooth. Spread the mixture in an even layer on the puff pastry, leaving a 1-inch (2.5 cm) border at the edges. Sprinkle the blueberries evenly on top.

4 Starting on one long end, gently roll the puff pastry into a log. Slice the log into eight equal pieces, and place them on the baking sheet. (If the pinwheels are soft and difficult to slice, place the roll in the fridge for 10 minutes before slicing.) Leave 1 to 2 inches (2.5 to 5 cm) of space between each of the pieces because they will spread as they bake.

5 Whisk the egg with 1 tablespoon of water in a small bowl, and lightly brush the top of each pinwheel with the egg wash.

6 Bake for 20 to 25 minutes, until golden brown.

7 Let cool completely before serving.

Peanut Butter Banana Pinwheels

1 Preheat the oven to 400°F (200°C). Line a baking sheet with parchment paper.

2 Dust a work surface with flour and then unfold the puff pastry sheet onto the surface.

3 Spread the peanut butter in an even layer on the puff pastry, leaving a 1-inch (2.5 cm) border at the edges. Spread the banana slices evenly over the peanut butter. Sprinkle the cinnamon evenly over the bananas.

4 Starting on one long end, gently roll the puff pastry into a log. Slice the log into eight equal pieces, and place them on the baking sheet. (If the pinwheels are soft and difficult to slice, place the roll in the fridge for 10 minutes before slicing.) Leave 1 to 2 inches (2.5 to 5 cm) of space between each of the pieces because they will spread as they bake.

5 Whisk the egg with 1 tablespoon of water in a small bowl, and lightly brush the top of each pinwheel with the egg wash.

6 Bake for 20 to 25 minutes, until golden brown.

7 Let cool completely before serving.

garlic Bread Bites

prep **15 minutes** / cook **15 minutes** / makes **40 bites**

1¾ cups (228 g) all-purpose flour (plus more for dusting)

1 cup (240 g) plain whole milk Greek yogurt

1 tablespoon baking powder

¼ teaspoon garlic powder

1 teaspoon salt

4 tablespoons unsalted butter, melted

2 garlic cloves, minced

1 teaspoon Italian seasoning

2 tablespoons grated Parmesan

These bites of garlic bread are light and airy; they're the perfect filling snack! Their soft and pillowy texture makes them easy for little ones to break down and eat. And the best part is, there's no need for yeast—just mix, knead, roll, and bake!

1 Preheat the oven to 375°F (190°C). Line a baking sheet with parchment paper.

2 Mix the flour, yogurt, baking powder, garlic powder, and salt in a large bowl until a dough forms.

3 Dust a work surface with flour. Turn out the dough onto the surface, and knead until smooth and elastic, 5 to 8 minutes. Cut it into four equal pieces.

4 Roll each piece into a 10-inch (25 cm) log, and slice into ten 1-inch (2.5 cm) pieces (see Tip 1). Place the pieces onto the baking pan.

5 Mix the butter, garlic, and Italian seasoning in a small bowl. Brush the butter sauce on top of each dough piece, fully coating all the edges.

6 Bake for 15 minutes, until the edges are lightly golden (see Tip 2).

7 Remove from the oven and immediately top with Parmesan. Let cool before serving.

Storage

Store in an airtight container at room temperature for up to 2 days or in the fridge for up to 5 days. To freeze, store in a freezer-safe airtight container for up to 3 months. Reheat in the microwave for 15 to 20 seconds, until warmed through.

Tips

1. You can shape a few of the dough pieces into mini logs (combine two small 1-inch/2.5 cm pieces) to make larger bites or breadsticks for your little one.

2. You can shake the pan halfway through for even browning, but it's not necessary.

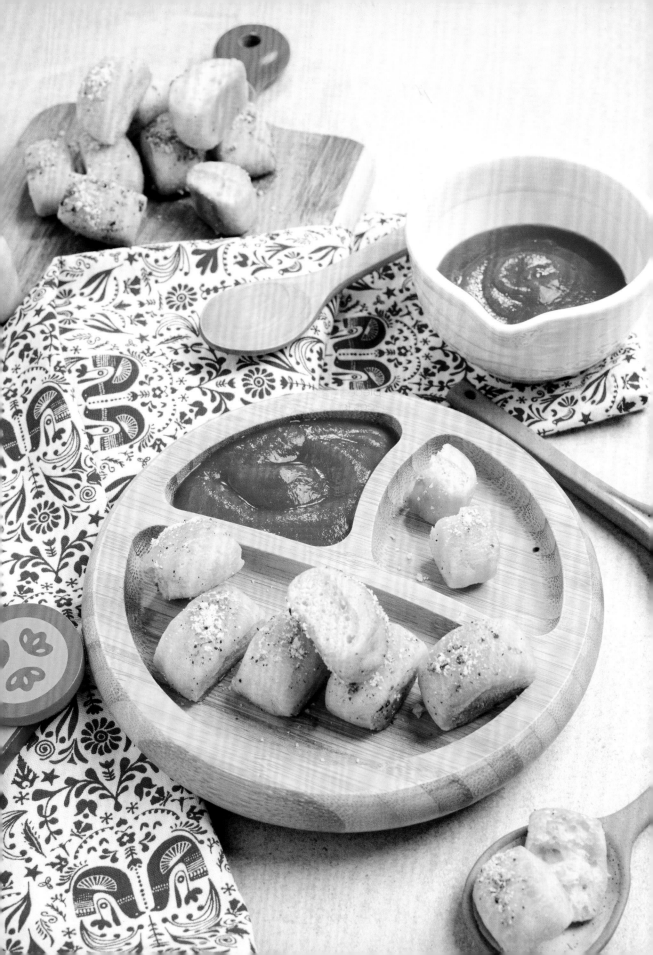

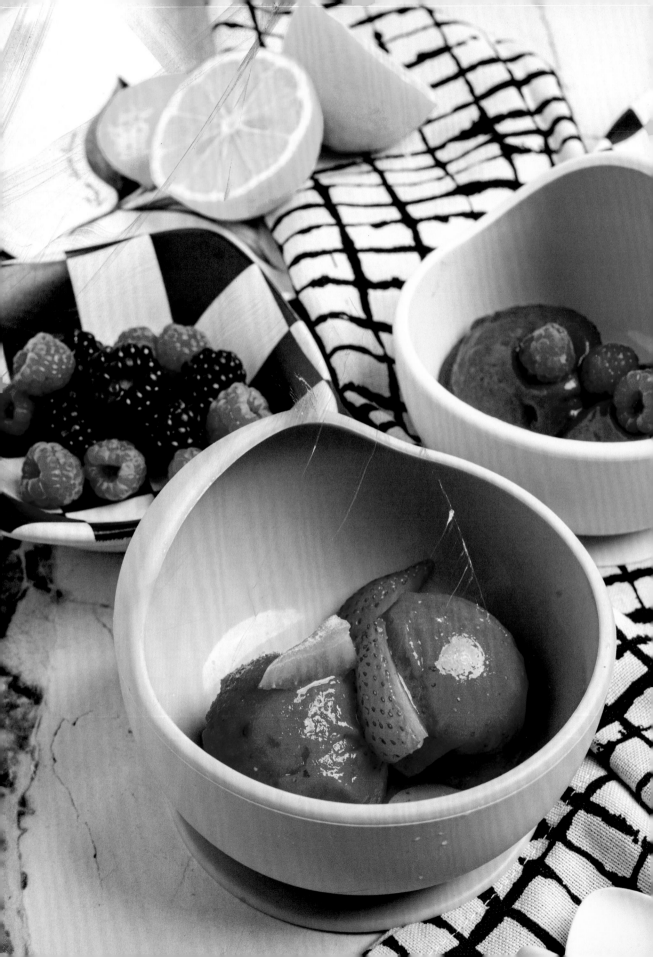

Fruity Sorbet & "Nice" Cream

prep **10 minutes** / serves **2 adults & 2 children**

Strawberry Lemon Sorbet

1 pound (454 g) frozen strawberries (about 3 cups)

¼ cup (60 ml) fresh lemon juice

1 to 2 tablespoons maple syrup (optional, see Tip 1)

Chocolate Banana "Nice" Cream

2 large ripe bananas, peeled, sliced, and frozen

2 tablespoons unsweetened cocoa powder (see Tip 2)

1 tablespoon natural peanut butter

2 tablespoons coconut milk (or milk of choice)

1 teaspoon ground cinnamon

It's amazing how much sweetness natural fruits can add to a recipe. These frozen treats are perfect for the summertime but can be enjoyed all year round. They're made with simple, fresh ingredients that come together quickly in the blender for a creamy, sweet treat.

1 Add the ingredients for your preferred flavor to a food processor, and blend until smooth. Scrape down the sides as needed to incorporate. Add a little more liquid in small increments as needed if it is difficult to blend.

2 Serve immediately for a soft-serve texture. If you prefer a thicker consistency, pour the mixture into a 9 × 5-inch (23 × 13 cm) loaf pan or airtight container and place in the freezer for 15 to 20 minutes to firm up.

3 Use an ice cream scoop to scoop and serve.

Storage

Store in a freezer-safe airtight container in the freezer for up to 1 month.

Tips

1. Remove baby's portion, and add maple syrup for some added sweetness for the rest of the family.

2. If you prefer to avoid serving cocoa powder to your little one, replace it with 1 extra tablespoon of peanut butter for peanut butter "nice" cream, or omit it for classic banana "nice" cream.

Blueberry Almond Scones

prep **5 minutes** / cook **20 minutes** / makes **8 scones**

1½ cups (150 g) almond flour

1 teaspoon baking powder

2 tablespoons unsalted butter, melted and cooled

2 tablespoons maple syrup

1 teaspoon vanilla extract

⅓ cup (50 g) blueberries (see Tip 1)

These scones are soft and chewy and made with simple ingredients. They don't have a typical scone texture; instead, they have the perfect soft texture for little ones to easily break down and eat. They have a nutty flavor from the almond flour and are bursting with blueberry pieces in every bite!

1 Preheat the oven to 350°F (180°C). Line a baking sheet with parchment paper.

2 Stir together the almond flour and baking powder in a large bowl.

3 Add the butter, maple syrup, and vanilla extract, and mix until combined. The dough may seem crumbly at first, but keep mixing (using your hands if necessary) until it comes together.

4 Gently fold in the blueberries, so they don't burst. The mixture should be slightly moist.

5 Transfer the dough to the baking sheet, and flatten it into a disc about 6 inches (15 cm) in diameter. Use a pizza slicer or a knife to cut the dough into eight wedges, keeping the circular shape.

6 Bake for 15 to 20 minutes, until the edges are golden.

7 Let the scones cool completely before separating and removing them from the baking sheet (see Tip 2).

Storage

Store in an airtight container at room temperature for up to 2 days or in the refrigerator for up to 5 days. The scones will soften in texture with moisture from the blueberries but will still have the same taste. To freeze, store in a freezer-safe bag with most of the air removed for up to 2 months. Reheat in a 250°F (120°C) oven until warmed through.

Tips

1. The blueberries in these scones are cooked and soft, but whole, uncooked blueberries are a choking hazard. When serving fresh blueberries to babies or young toddlers, quarter or smash them into discs to eliminate roundness.

2. Don't remove the scones from the baking sheet until they are completely cool so they don't fall apart. They will be soft in texture from the blueberries but will firm up and darken as they cool.

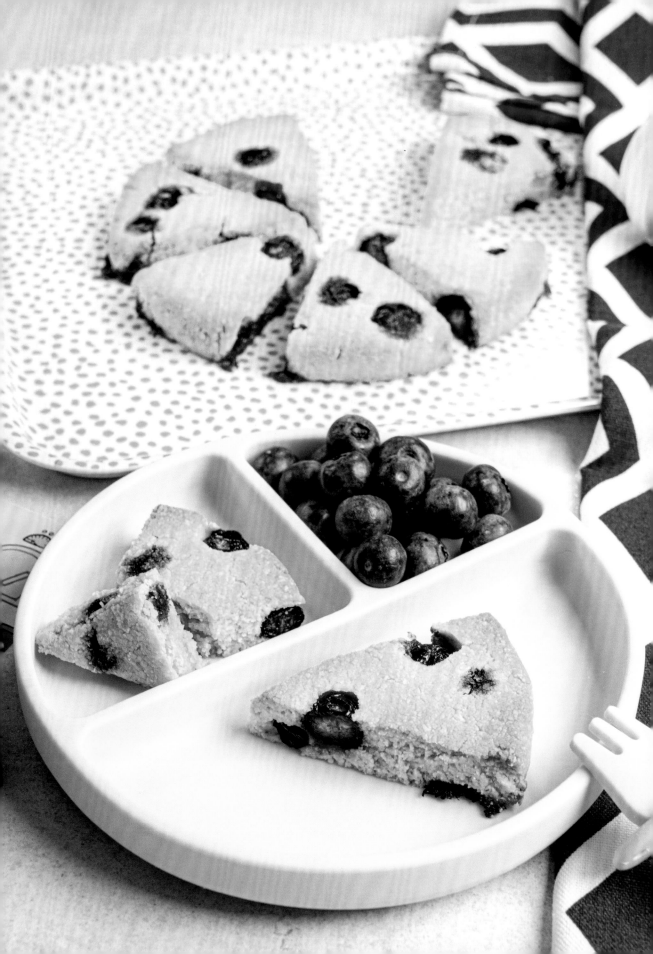

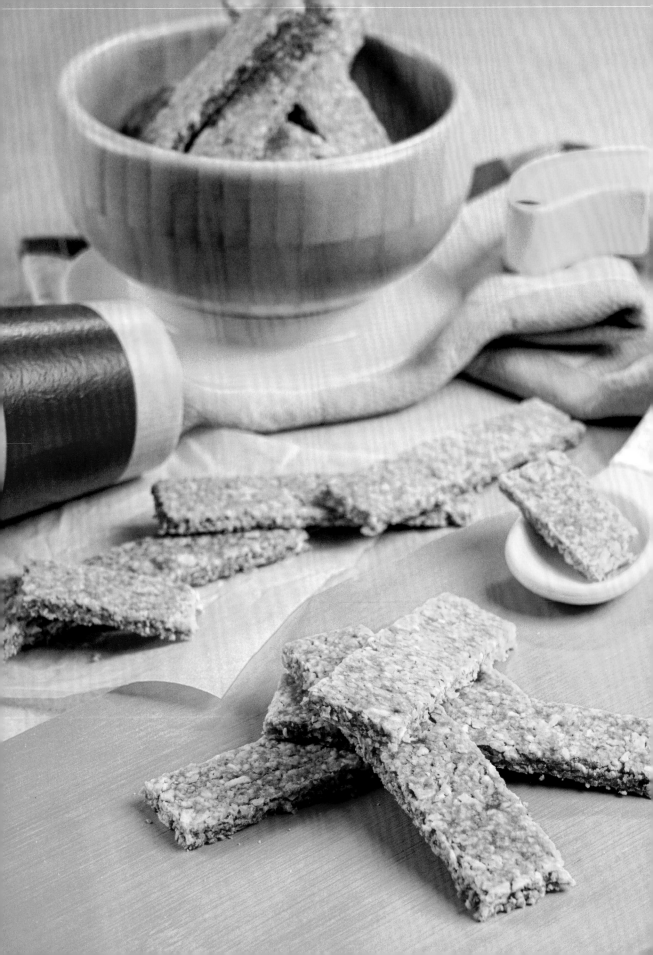

Banana Teething Biscuits

prep **10 minutes** / cook **10 minutes** / makes **24 biscuits**

1½ cups (135 g) old-fashioned rolled oats

⅓ cup (80 g) mashed ripe banana (from 1 small banana)

1 tablespoon mild-tasting oil

¼ teaspoon ground cinnamon

¼ teaspoon ground ginger

These banana biscuits are perfect for soothing little gums! They are naturally sweetened with banana and have the perfect soft texture for babies to gnaw on. I created these biscuits with my teething son in mind, but I love dunking them into peanut butter or hazelnut spread for myself!

1 Preheat the oven to 350°F (180°C).

2 Add the oats to a food processor or blender, and blend to form a flour-like texture. Transfer to a large bowl.

3 Add the banana, oil, cinnamon, and ginger to the bowl, and mix with a fork to form a dough (see Tip 1).

4 Place the dough between two sheets of parchment paper, and roll it out into a thin 7 × 10-inch (18 × 25 cm) rectangle. Use a pizza slicer or a knife to slice the dough into 24 rectangular sticks. Transfer the parchment paper to a baking sheet.

5 Bake for 10 minutes, or until the tops are firm to the touch.

6 Let cool completely before separating the biscuits. They will continue to firm up as they cool (see Tip 2).

Storage

Store in an airtight container at room temperature for up to 4 days or in the freezer for up to 2 months. Thaw at room temperature before serving.

Tips

1. Stir a teaspoon of ground flaxseeds into the dough mixture for a nutritional boost.
2. Pop these into the freezer for a few minutes to cool for a cold treat for your teething baby to gnaw on and soothe those gums!

Raspberry Bliss Balls

prep **10 minutes** / chill **15 minutes** / makes **16 balls**

1¼ cups (113 g) old-fashioned rolled oats

½ cup (40 g) desiccated coconut, plus more to coat

1 cup (120 g) frozen raspberries

¼ cup (50 g) raisins

These bliss balls are an easy, no-bake snack option. They come together with only four ingredients and are naturally sweetened with raspberries and raisins. They're also free from many top allergens, making them a great snack for school or day care.

1 Add the ingredients to a food processor (not a blender; see Tip 1), and blend to combine.

2 Scoop out tablespoon-sized portions of the mixture, and roll them into balls (see Tip 2). Wet your hands as you roll because the mixture will be sticky.

3 Roll the balls in desiccated coconut to coat, and transfer them to a plate.

4 Place the balls in the fridge for at least 15 minutes to firm up.

Storage

Store in an airtight container in the refrigerator for up to 2 days. To freeze, store in a freezer-safe bag for up to 1 month. Thaw at room temperature before serving.

Tips

1. It's important to use a food processor for this recipe because a blender will not be powerful enough to break down the mixture without added moisture.
2. If preparing this for a young baby, make the bliss balls large (bigger than baby's mouth) or shape them into finger-length strips.

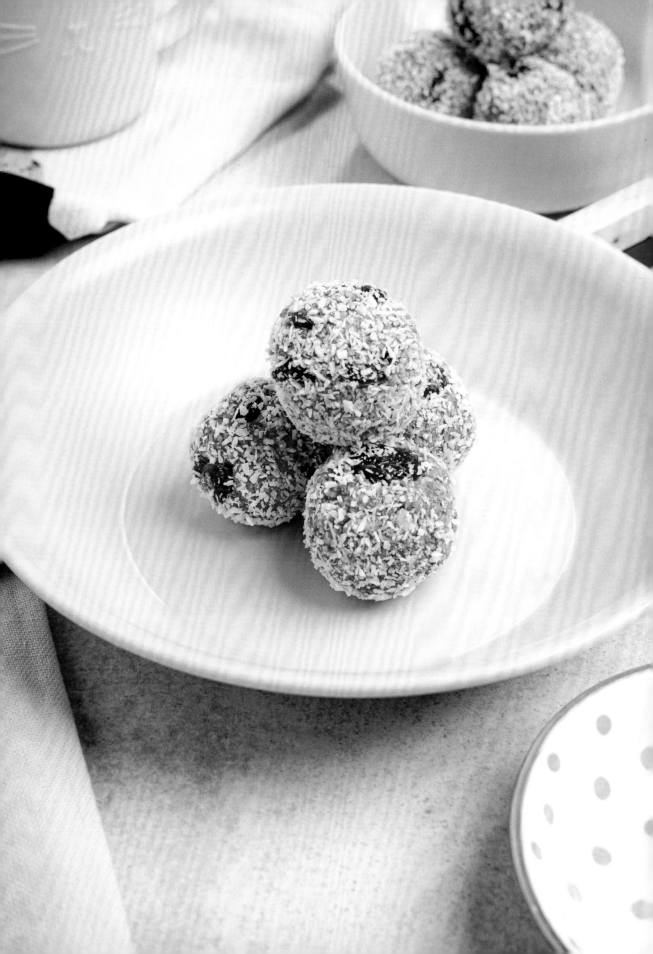

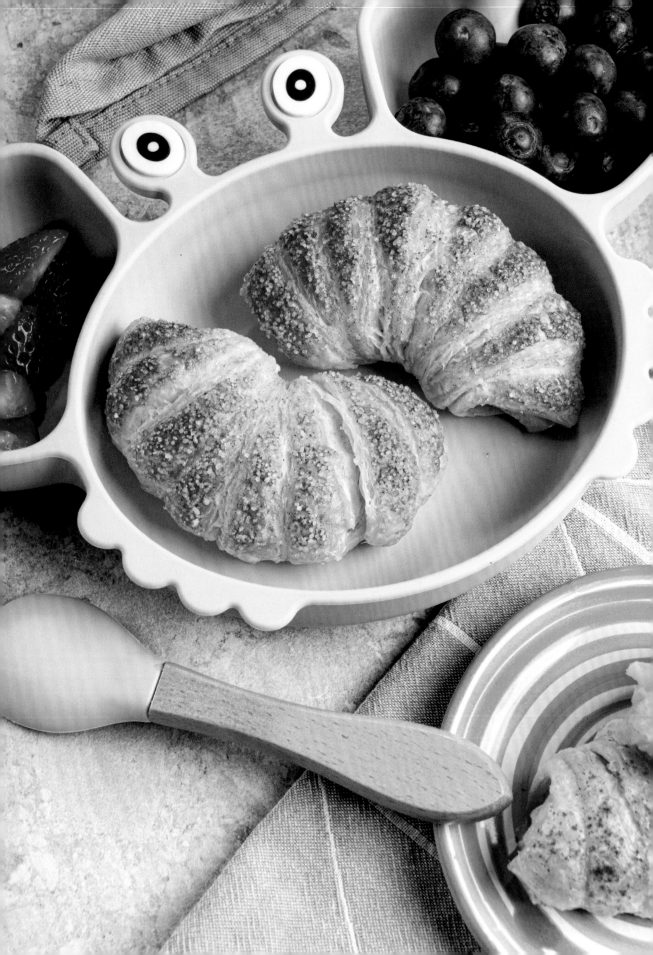

DF NF V

Apple Croissant Pastries

prep **10 minutes** / cook **25 minutes** / makes **10 mini croissants**

Apple Pastries

All-purpose flour, for dusting

1 sheet (245 g) puff pastry, thawed

1 large apple (preferably Honeycrisp, see Tip 1)

1 egg (see Tip 2)

Cinnamon Sugar Coating

2 tablespoons sugar

1 teaspoon ground cinnamon

These apple croissant pastries combine the buttery flakiness of puff pastry with sweet, crisp apples. As they bake, the apples soften and become tender, creating a juicy filling and a melt-in-your-mouth treat the whole family will love!

1 Preheat the oven to 350°F (180°C). Line a baking sheet with parchment paper.

2 Dust a work surface with flour and then unfold the puff pastry sheet onto the surface.

3 Lightly roll out the puff pastry sheet to smooth it out, and slice it into 20 thin strips along the long end.

4 Slice the apple into five thin rings and use a teaspoon to cut out the core in the center. Slice the apple rings in half to form two moon shapes.

5 Starting on one end of the apple, wrap a strip of puff pastry around the wedge. Add another strip and continue to wrap until the apple is fully covered. Press down on the covered apple to make sure that the puff pastry is tightly secured onto the apple, and place it on the baking sheet. Repeat for the rest of the apple wedges.

6 Whisk the egg with 1 tablespoon of water in a small bowl, and lightly brush the top of each croissant with the egg wash.

7 Mix the sugar and cinnamon in a small bowl. Sprinkle the top of each croissant generously with cinnamon sugar (see Tip 3).

8 Bake for 25 minutes, or until golden brown.

9 Let cool completely before serving.

Storage

Store in an airtight container in the refrigerator for up to 3 days. To freeze, store in a freezer-safe bag for up to 1 month. Reheat in a 350°F (180°C) oven for 10 minutes, or until warmed through.

Tips

1. If you prefer to peel the apple, you can do this before slicing it into rings. If you choose not to peel, the skin will soften while baking.

2. Egg-free? Swap the egg with melted butter or oil.

3. If preparing these for a baby, omit the cinnamon sugar and sprinkle with a little ground cinnamon instead.

Cream Cheese Crackers

prep **10 minutes** / cook **18 minutes** / serves **1 adult & 2 children**

¾ cup (98 g) all-purpose flour, plus more for dusting

¼ cup (55 g) cream cheese, cold and cubed

3 tablespoons unsalted butter, cold and cubed

My son Myles loves helping out in the kitchen, and this is the perfect recipe for him to help me with. The cracker dough comes together with just three ingredients, is easy to work with, and requires no kneading. Myles loves cutting out his crackers in fun shapes, and the batches we make never last long!

1 Preheat the oven to 350°F (180°C).

2 Mix the flour, cream cheese, and butter in a medium bowl. Use your fingers to work the butter and cream cheese into the flour to form a dough.

3 Flour a sheet of parchment paper, place the dough on the parchment paper, and roll it out into an 8-inch (20 cm) square, about ⅛ inch (3 mm) thick (see Tip 1). If the dough is a little sticky, roll it between two sheets of parchment paper.

4 Use a pizza slicer or a knife to slice the dough into 1 × 2-inch (2.5 × 5 cm) crackers. Use a fork to poke holes in the crackers for ventilation. Transfer the parchment paper to a baking sheet.

5 Bake for 15 to 18 minutes, until the edges are slightly brown (see Tip 2).

6 Let cool completely before serving.

Storage

Store in an airtight container at room temperature for up to 2 days. The crackers will soften in texture the longer they are stored.

Tips

1. For softer crackers, roll out the dough to ¼ inch (6 mm) thick.

2. If preparing these for a baby, bake them for just 10 to 12 minutes so they break down more easily in the mouth.

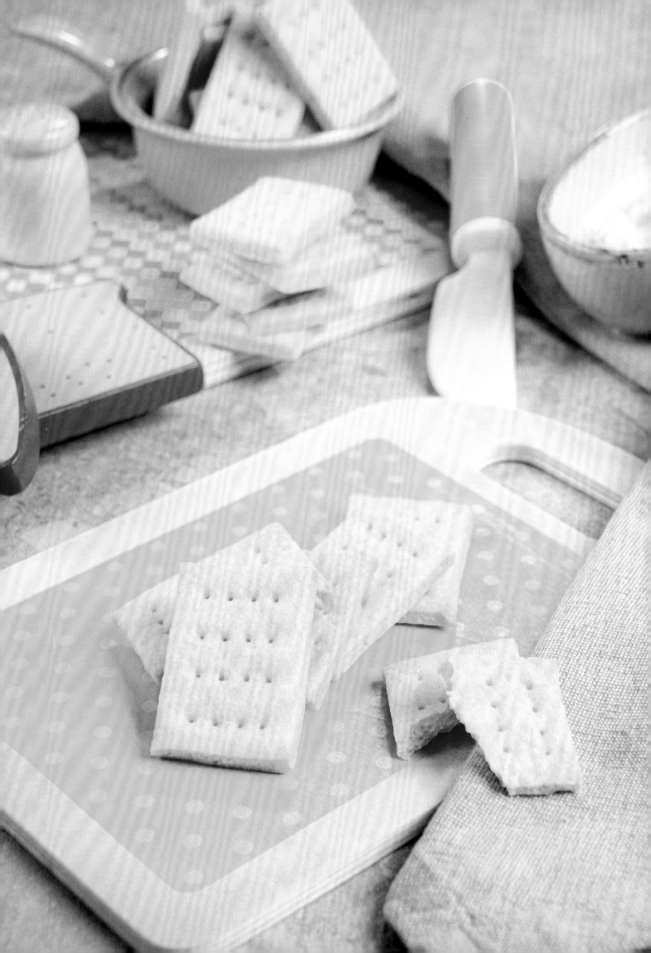

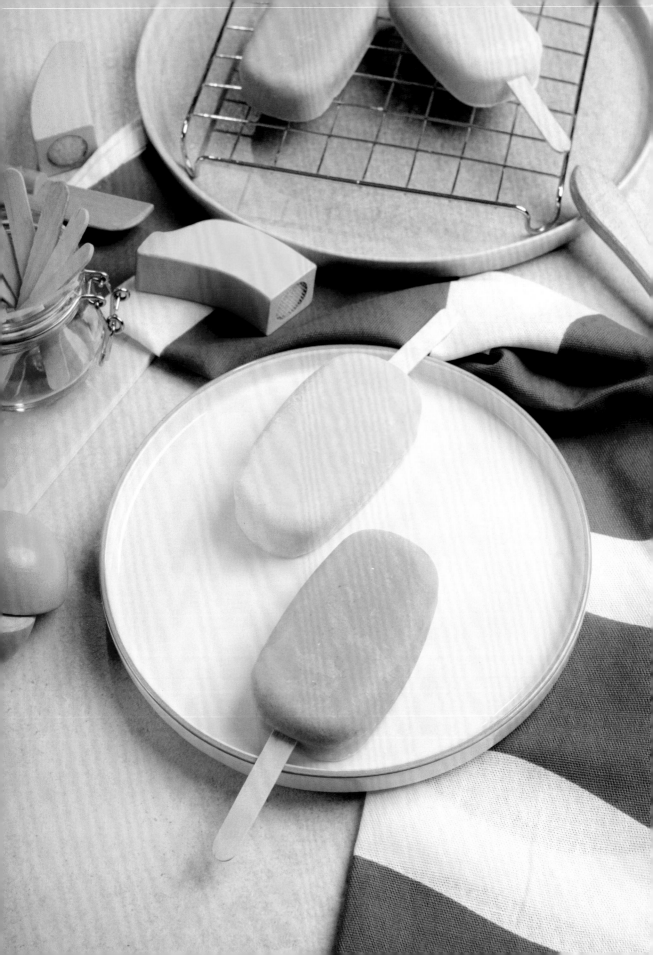

Fruity Smoothie Pops

prep **5 minutes** / freeze **4 hours** / makes **9 to 12 mini pops**

These fruit-rich smoothie pops are a refreshing sweet treat that can be enjoyed all year long. They are naturally sweetened with fruits and can be customized with add-ins for fun flavor combinations!

EF **GF** **NF** **V**

Spinach Banana Smoothie Pops

2 large ripe bananas, thinly sliced

1 cup (240 g) plain whole milk Greek yogurt (see Tip 1)

½ cup (30 g) spinach, tightly packed

⅛ teaspoon ground cinnamon

Spinach Banana Smoothie Pops

1 Add the ingredients to a blender, and blend until completely smooth.

2 Pour the mixture into mini silicone popsicle molds (see Tip 2).

3 Freeze for at least 4 hours.

EF **GF** **NF** **V**

Mango Smoothie Pops

2 cups (280 g) fresh or frozen mango chunks

1 cup (240 g) plain whole milk Greek yogurt (see Tip 1)

1 to 2 teaspoons maple syrup (optional)

Mango Smoothie Pops

1 Add the ingredients to a blender, and blend until smooth. If it is difficult to blend, add a few splashes of milk to the blender, and scrape down the sides as needed.

2 Pour the mixture into mini silicone popsicle molds (see Tip 2).

3 Freeze for at least 4 hours.

Storage

Transfer the smoothie pops to a freezer-safe airtight container to prevent freezer burn, and store in the freezer for up to 3 months.

Tips

1. Dairy-free? Replace the yogurt with unsweetened applesauce.
2. Use small popsicle molds so that the pops are a manageable size for a young baby. Silicone molds are my favorite for pops that literally "pop" right out!

Zucchini Bites

prep **10 minutes** / cook **18 minutes** / makes **15 to 18 mini bites**

1 large zucchini
¼ cup (28 g) shredded cheddar
1 egg (see Tip 1)
3 tablespoons oat flour (see Tip 2)
¼ teaspoon onion powder
¼ teaspoon salt (optional)

Zucchini can be pretty bland on its own, but the cheesy taste of these bites makes for a great, filling snack. They are so simple to make, and once you try one, it'll be hard to stop snacking on them!

1 Preheat the oven to 350°F (180°C). Line a baking sheet with parchment paper.

2 Use a cheese grater to grate the zucchini, using the smallest holes for a smoother texture. You can leave on the skin for more nutrients. Measure 1 cup (220 g) packed grated zucchini.

3 Use a cheesecloth, a clean kitchen towel, or your hands to squeeze out all of the excess moisture. You should have about ½ cup (90 g) of zucchini.

4 Place the zucchini in a medium bowl along with the cheddar, egg, flour, onion powder, and salt (if using). Mix until well combined.

5 Scoop out teaspoon-sized portions of the mixture, and place on the baking sheet. Press down to flatten them to about ¼ inch (6 mm) thick.

6 Bake for 15 to 18 minutes, until golden around the edges.

7 Let cool completely before serving.

Storage

Store in an airtight container in the fridge for up to 3 days. To freeze, store in a freezer-safe bag with most of the air removed for up to 3 months. To reheat, microwave for 10 to 15 seconds, until warmed through.

Tips

1. Egg-free? Swap the egg with a flax egg (see page 55).
2. To make your own oat flour, blend ½ cup (45 g) of dry old-fashioned rolled oats in a high-powered blender or a food processor until very fine. You can also replace it with a different type of flour.

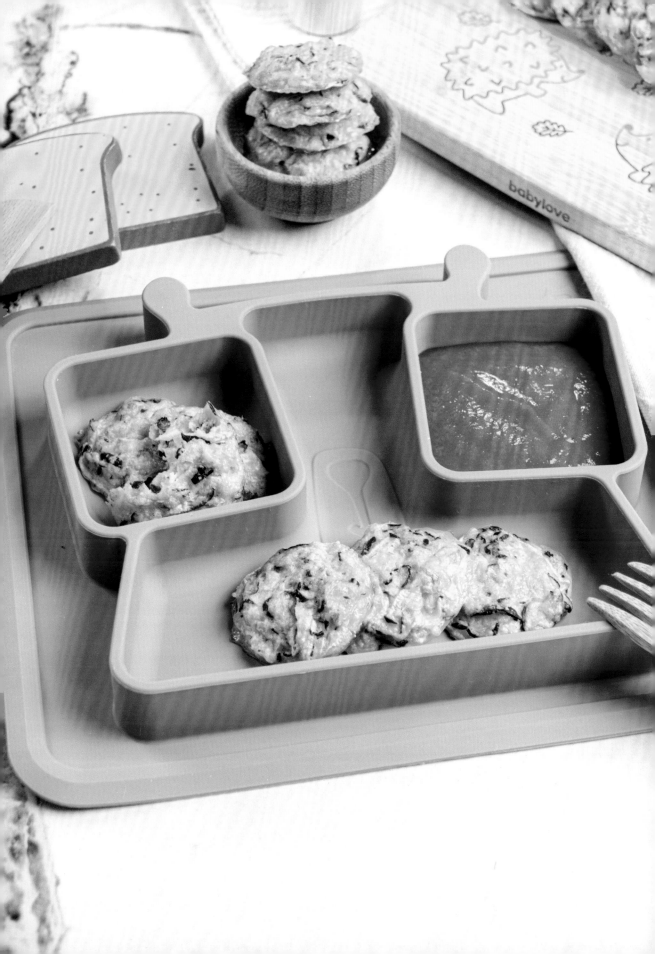

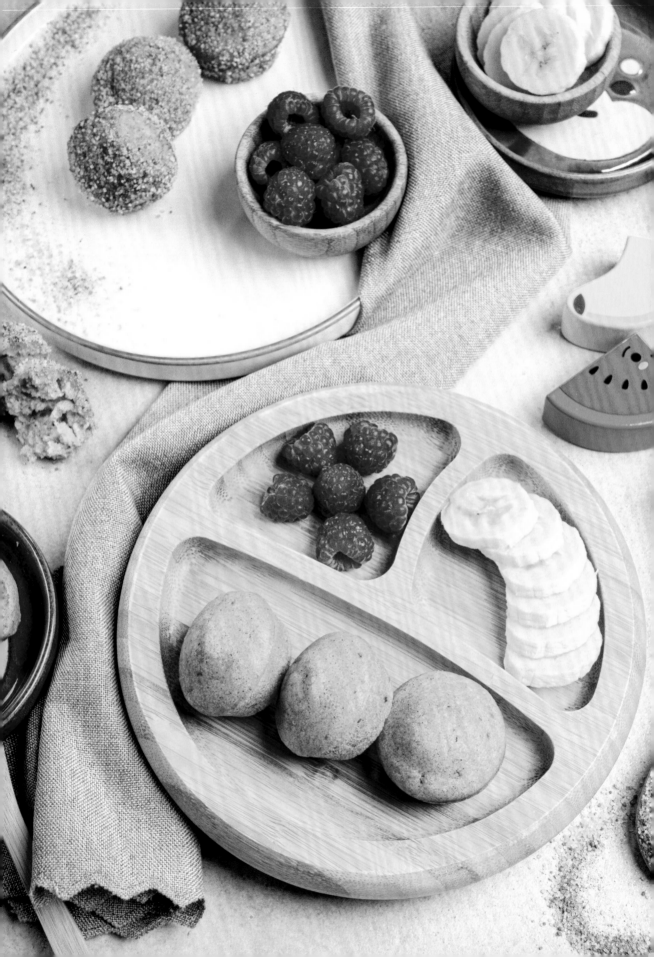

Cinnamon Apple Doughnut Muffins

prep **10 minutes** / cook **15 minutes** / makes **24 mini muffins**

½ cup (125 g) unsweetened applesauce

⅓ cup (80 ml) milk

1 egg (see Tip 1)

3 tablespoons mild-tasting oil

3 tablespoons maple syrup

1 cup (130 g) all-purpose flour

2 teaspoons baking powder

1 teaspoon ground cinnamon

Cinnamon Sugar Coating (optional)

2 tablespoons sugar

1 teaspoon ground cinnamon

2 tablespoons unsalted butter, melted

These cinnamon apple muffins are a cross between mini muffins and doughnut holes. They have a mini muffin shape and a soft and fluffy doughnut texture and are coated in cinnamon goodness.

1 Preheat the oven to 350°F (180°C).

2 Whisk together the applesauce, milk, egg, oil, and maple syrup in a large bowl until smooth.

3 Add the flour, baking powder, and cinnamon, and mix until just combined.

4 Place tablespoon-sized portions of batter into a 24-cup silicone mini-muffin pan (see Tip 2).

5 Bake for 15 minutes, or until a toothpick inserted into the center of a muffin comes out clean.

6 Let the muffins cool completely before removing from the pan.

7 For an optional cinnamon coating, mix together the sugar and cinnamon in a small bowl. Lightly brush the muffins with melted butter and dip them into the cinnamon-sugar mixture to coat, shaking off any excess (see Tip 3).

Storage

Store in an airtight container at room temperature for up to 2 days or in the fridge for up to 5 days. To freeze, store in a freezer-safe bag with most of the air removed for up to 3 months. To reheat, microwave for 20 to 30 seconds, until warmed through.

Tips

1. Egg-free? Swap the egg with a liquid egg substitute like JUST Egg.
2. If you don't have a silicone mini-muffin pan, you can use a metal 24-cup mini-muffin pan. If using a metal mini-muffin pan, be sure to grease the pan with cooking spray so the muffins won't stick.
3. If you prefer, sprinkle the cinnamon sugar on top of the muffins before baking.

Strawberry Oat Cookies

prep **8 minutes** / cook **12 minutes** / makes **15 cookies**

1 large overripe banana

3 tablespoons natural peanut butter (see Tip 1)

1 cup (90 g) old-fashioned rolled oats

½ cup (90 g) finely chopped strawberries

¼ cup (43 g) chocolate chips (optional)

These strawberry and oat cookies have the perfect soft texture for babies and are naturally sweetened with fruits. They're a great way of getting in a serving of oats, and the combination of oats, peanut butter, and fruit makes for a balanced snack!

1 Preheat the oven to 350°F (180°C). Line a large baking sheet with parchment paper.

2 Mash the banana in a large bowl until smooth. Add the peanut butter and oats, and stir to combine.

3 Gently fold in the strawberries and chocolate chips (if using; see Tip 2).

4 Scoop heaping tablespoon–sized portions of the mixture onto the baking sheet, and press down on each portion to flatten into thin rounds.

5 Bake for 10 to 12 minutes, until firm to the touch.

6 Let cool completely before serving.

Storage

Store in an airtight container at room temperature for up to 2 days or in the refrigerator for up to 5 days. To freeze, store in a freezer-safe bag for up to 2 months. To reheat, microwave for 10 to 15 seconds, until warmed through. You can also let the cookies thaw completely at room temperature for 1 or 2 hours.

Tips

1. Nut-free? Swap the peanut butter with a seed-based spread like sunflower seed butter, or omit it completely.

2. Feel free to stir in more add-ins like finely chopped nuts, fruits, or more chocolate chips! You also can set aside some of the mixture for your baby and stir in more add-ins for everyone else.

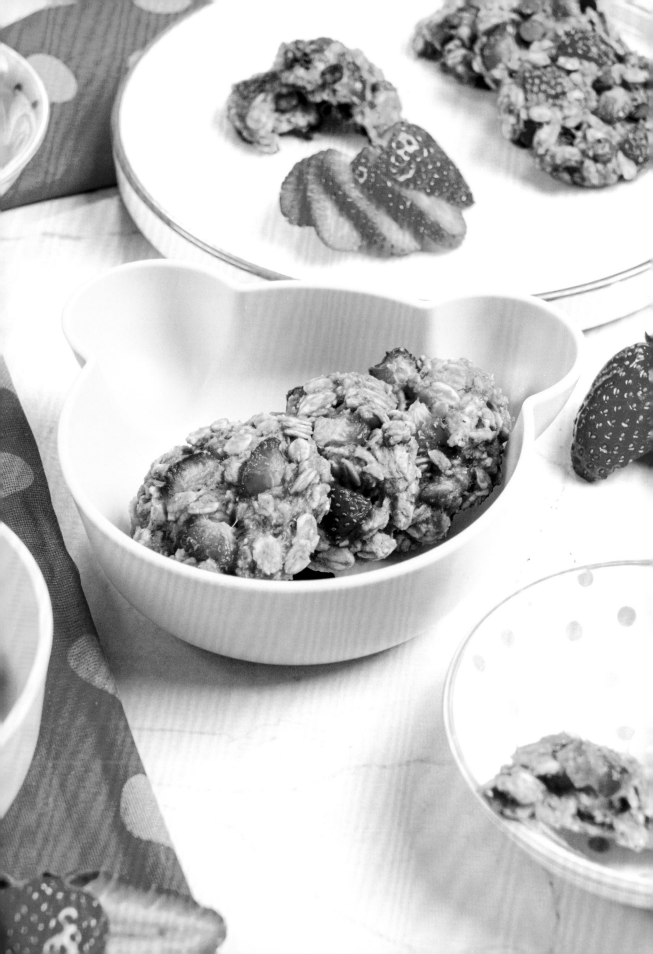

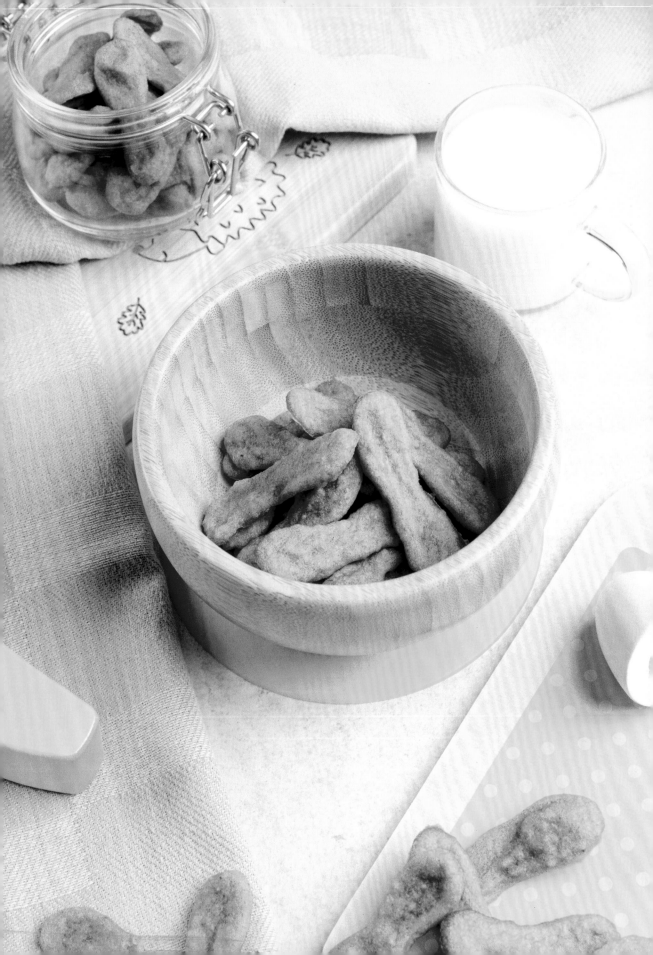

Apple Banana Strips

prep **5 minutes** / cook **18 minutes** / makes **about 24 strips**

½ cup (45 g) old-fashioned rolled oats

¼ cup (63 g) unsweetened applesauce (see Tip 1)

¼ cup (63 g) mashed overripe banana (from 1 small banana)

1 egg yolk (see Tip 2)

2 teaspoons mild-tasting oil

½ teaspoon baking powder

¼ teaspoon ground cinnamon

These apple and banana strips are the perfect snack for tiny taste buds! They're naturally sweetened with fruits and easy for little ones to grasp. The flavor profiles are customizable by swapping in your favorite mashed fruits.

1 Preheat the oven to 350°F (180°C). Line a baking sheet with parchment paper.

2 Blend all the ingredients together in a blender until smooth.

3 Pour the mixture into a piping bag or ziplock plastic bag with one corner tip cut off.

4 Pipe out 2 × ½-inch (5 × 1 cm) strips onto the baking sheet.

5 Bake for 10 minutes, or until the edges are slightly golden.

6 Turn off the oven and let the puffs sit inside for an additional 5 to 8 minutes, until the edges begin to brown slightly. They will continue to bake from the residual oven heat.

7 Let cool before serving.

Storage

Store in an airtight container at room temperature for up to 5 days. To freeze, store in a freezer-safe bag for up to 3 months. To reheat, microwave for 10 to 15 seconds, or until warmed through. You can also let the strips thaw completely at room temperature for about 1 hour.

Tips

1. Want to switch up the flavor? Swap the applesauce and mashed banana with equal parts of different pureed or mashed fruits!

2. Egg-free? Replace the egg yolk with 2 tablespoons of flax egg mixture (see page 55) or 2 tablespoons of a liquid egg substitute like JUST Egg.

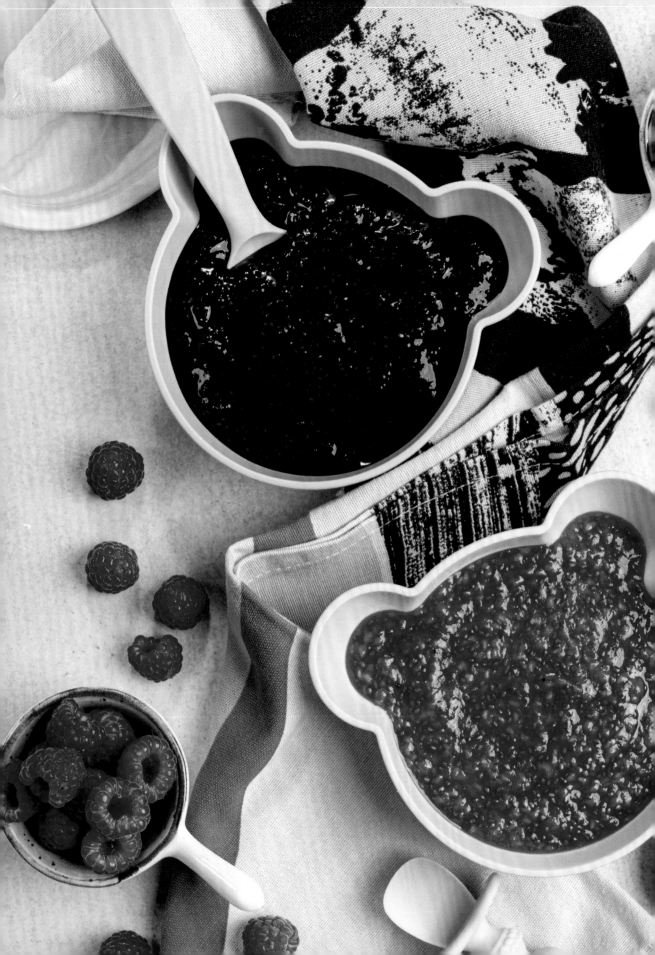

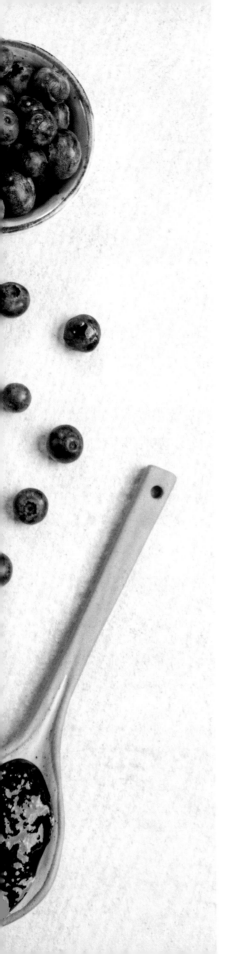

Sides, Spreads & Dips

It can be so hard to find spreads and dips that are suitable for babies but don't contain a ton of sugar and additives. It can also be tough to figure out how to make flavorful veggie sides that are baby-friendly and can be adjusted to taste for everyone else. This chapter contains some homemade jams, toppings, naturally flavored yogurts, and tasty veggies to pair with your favorite family meals.

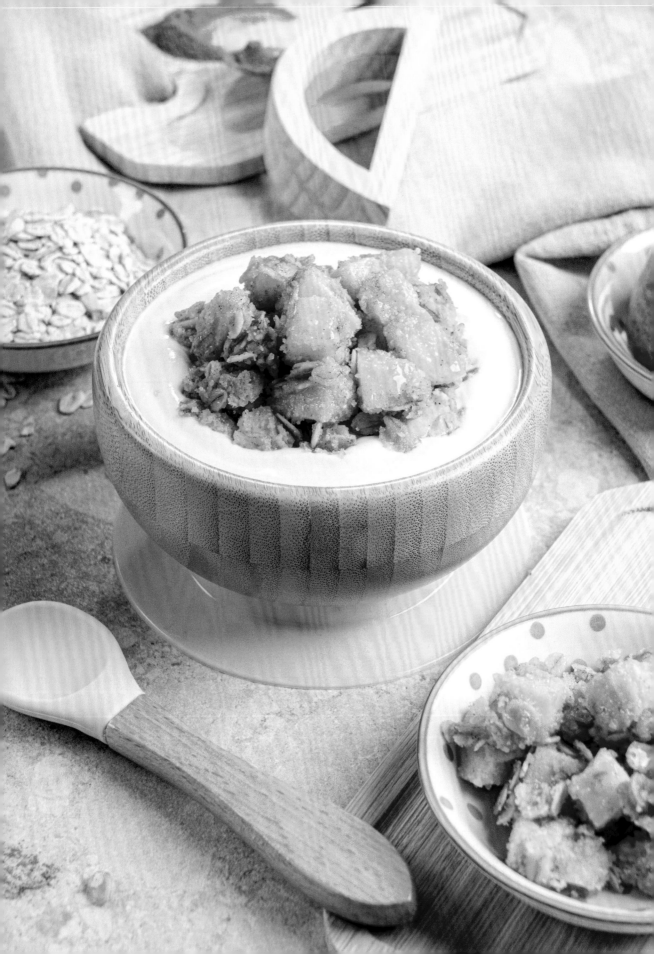

Stovetop Apple Crisp

prep **5 minutes** / cook **10 minutes** / serves **1 adult & 1 child**

3 tablespoons unsalted butter, divided

½ cup (45 g) old-fashioned rolled oats

1 small apple (preferably Honeycrisp or Fuji, see Tip 1)

1 teaspoon ground cinnamon

3 tablespoons unsweetened applesauce, or 1 tablespoon maple syrup (see Tip 2)

¼ cup (25 g) almond flour (see Tip 3)

This quick and easy apple crisp is a delicious sweet treat to serve as a topping—or enjoy as is! I love scooping a big portion on top of a bowl of yogurt for breakfast. It comes together quickly on the stovetop, so there's no baking needed.

1 Melt 2 tablespoons of butter in a large pan over medium heat. Add the oats, and stir continuously until lightly toasted, 1 to 2 minutes. Watch carefully so that the oats don't burn. Remove the oats from the pan, and set aside.

2 Peel and chop the apple into small cubes.

3 Melt the remaining 1 tablespoon of butter in the pan, then reduce the heat to medium-low.

4 Add the apples to the pan along with the cinnamon. Stir well to coat the apples, then cook until softened, 2 to 3 minutes.

5 Add the applesauce, and stir to coat. Return the toasted oats to the pan, and stir.

6 Add the almond flour, and stir to combine.

7 Let cool before serving.

Storage

Store in an airtight container in the fridge for up to 5 days. Reheat in a medium pan over medium-low heat for 5 minutes, or microwave for 10 to 15 seconds. You can also serve this cold right from the fridge.

Tips

1. My favorite type of apple to use for this recipe is Honeycrisp. They are sweet and crisp and pair perfectly with cinnamon. If you're unable to find them, Fuji apples are another great sweet apple variety.

2. If preparing this for a baby, use unsweetened applesauce as the sweetener. It softens the crisp and is the perfect texture for babies. If you are preparing it for a toddler or an adult, use maple syrup as the sweetener.

3. Nut-free? Omit the almond flour completely for a similar taste.

Caramelized Bananas & Sautéed Pears

serves **1 adult & 1 child**

EF GF NF V

Caramelized Cinnamon Bananas

2 tablespoons unsalted butter (see Tip 1)

¼ teaspoon ground cinnamon

1 medium banana, sliced into ¼-inch (6 mm) slices

EF GF NF V

Sautéed Cinnamon Pears

2 medium ripe pears

1 tablespoon unsalted butter (see Tip 1)

½ teaspoon ground cinnamon

These warm, sweet, cinnamon-coated bananas and pears are the perfect toppings for pancakes, waffles, oatmeal, and yogurt. They're both also great served on a slice of toast for a quick lunch—or to snack on as is!

Caramelized Cinnamon Bananas

prep **3 minutes** / cook **6 minutes**

1 Melt the butter in a medium nonstick pan over medium heat. Stir in the cinnamon.

2 Add the banana to the pan in an even layer, and cook until caramelized, 2 to 3 minutes per side.

Sautéed Cinnamon Pears

prep **5 minutes** / cook **10 minutes**

1 Peel the pears, and chop them into small cubes (see Tip 2). You may leave the skin on if preferred.

2 Melt the butter in a medium pan over medium-low heat. Add the pears along with the cinnamon, and stir well to coat.

3 Reduce the heat to low, cover, and cook for 8 to 10 minutes, until the pears fully soften. Stir halfway through to prevent sticking.

Storage

Store in an airtight container in the fridge for up to 3 days. Reheat in a medium pan over medium-low heat for 5 minutes, or microwave for about 10 seconds. You can also serve both straight from the fridge.

Tips

1. Dairy-free? Swap the butter with coconut oil.
2. These diced pears are great for helping your baby develop and practice the pincer grasp. If your baby does not yet have the pincer grasp, slice the pears into thin wedges.

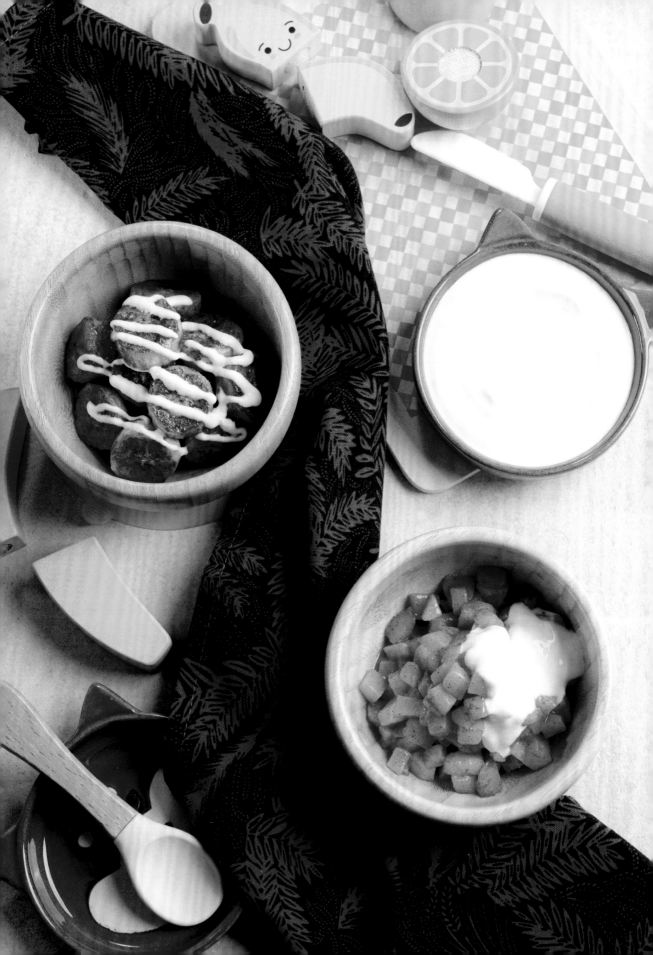

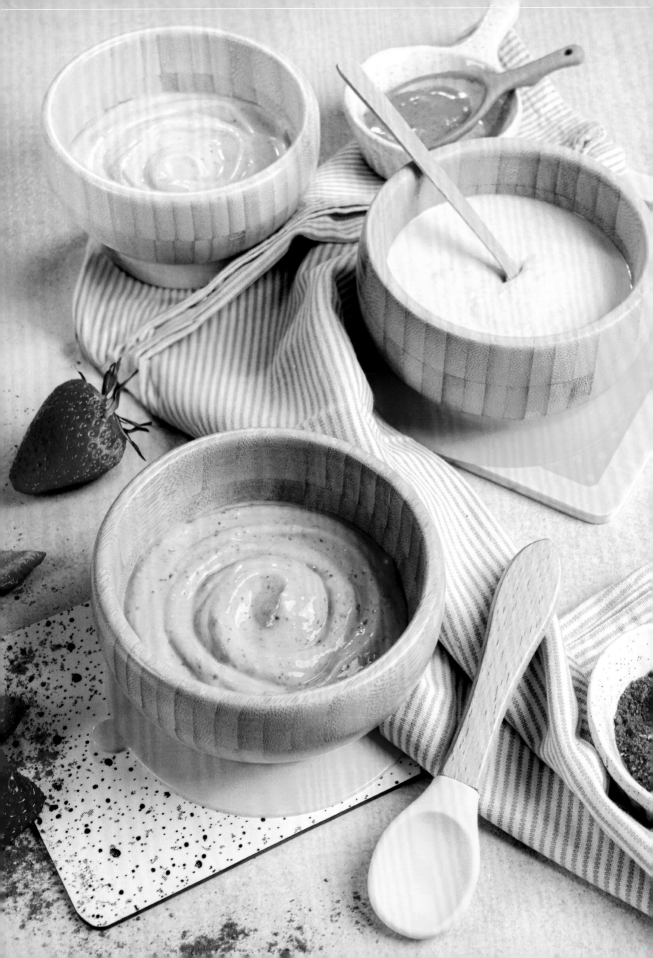

Flavored Yogurts

prep **5 minutes** / makes **½ cup (120 g; see Tip 1)**

I love taking a container of plain yogurt and jazzing it up with some fun flavors! It's easy to control the added sugar and customize the add-ins to your taste. Strawberry, pumpkin, and peanut butter yogurts are my boys' favorites, and this recipe works great with dairy-free yogurt as well.

1 For each flavored yogurt: Mix all the ingredients in a small bowl until smooth.

2 Taste, and adjust the sweetness as needed.

EF **GF** **NF** **V**

Strawberry Yogurt

- ½ cup (14 g) freeze-dried strawberries, crushed to a powder
- ½ cup (120 g) plain whole milk yogurt or Greek yogurt
- ¼ teaspoon vanilla extract

EF **GF** **NF** **V**

Pumpkin Yogurt

- ½ cup (120 g) plain whole milk yogurt or Greek yogurt
- 2 tablespoons pumpkin puree
- ¼ teaspoon pumpkin pie spice or ground cinnamon
- 1 teaspoon maple syrup (optional, see Tip 2)

EF **GF** **V**

Peanut Butter Yogurt

- ½ cup (120 g) plain whole milk yogurt or Greek yogurt
- 1 tablespoon natural peanut butter
- ½ teaspoon ground cinnamon
- 1 teaspoon maple syrup (optional, see Tip 2)

Storage

Store in an airtight container in the fridge. It will last as long as the date listed on the original yogurt container.

Tips

1. Feel free to double or triple the ingredients for a larger batch!
2. If preparing this for a young baby, replace the maple syrup with ½ mashed overripe banana.

guacamole

prep **5 minutes** / makes **1 cup (230 g)**

2 medium ripe avocados, pitted

1 small Roma tomato, finely diced

¼ cup (35 g) finely diced red onion (optional)

2 tablespoons finely chopped cilantro

¼ teaspoon garlic powder

1 tablespoon lime juice

¼ teaspoon salt (optional, see Tip)

Guacamole is a classic, and this is my go-to recipe for this fresh-tasting dip. I'm guilty of eating it by the spoonful, but I also love to spread it on a slice of toast for a filling lunch.

1 Scoop the avocado flesh into a medium bowl. Mash with a fork until smooth, leaving in some small chunks, if desired.

2 Add the tomato, onion (if using), cilantro, garlic powder, lime juice, and salt (if using), and mix until combined.

Storage

Store in an airtight container in the fridge for up to 2 days. It may begin to brown due to the natural oxidation of the avocados, but you can remove the top, browned layer, if needed, before serving.

Tip

- If preparing for a baby, remove baby's portion before stirring in ¼ teaspoon of salt for the rest of the family.

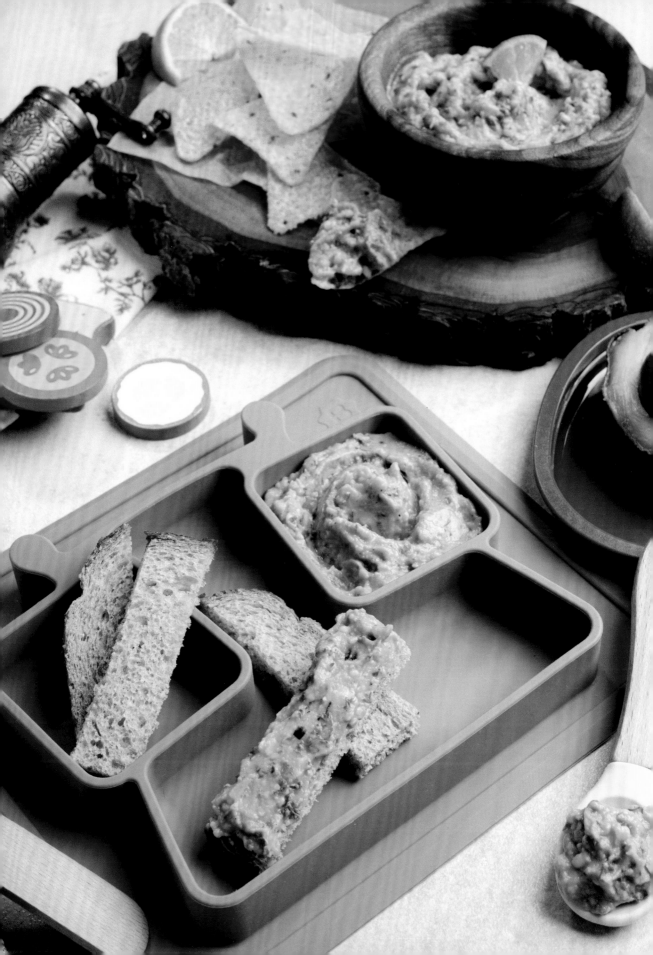

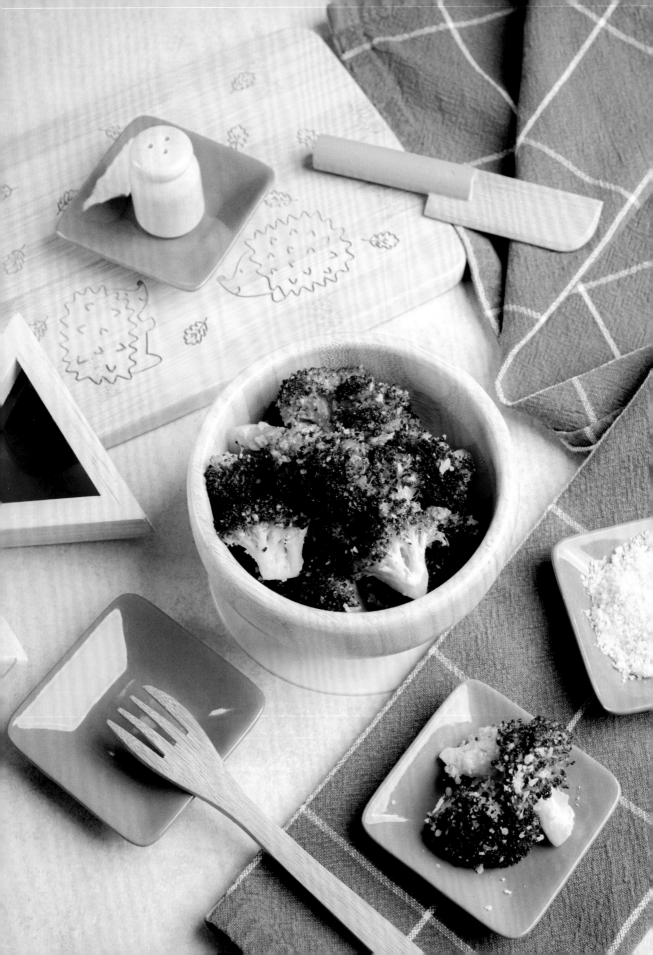

Parmesan-Roasted Broccoli

prep **5 minutes** / cook **18 minutes** / serves **2 adults & 1 child**

- 12 ounces (340 g) broccoli florets
- 2 tablespoons mild-tasting oil
- ¼ teaspoon garlic powder
- ¼ teaspoon black pepper
- 2 tablespoons grated Parmesan (see Tip 1)

Whenever I make this roasted broccoli for dinner, there isn't usually much left when it's time to serve it. As I'm prepping other items, I like to snack on this broccoli, and before I know it, the whole tray disappears. The combination of the slightly crisp edges and the Parmesan coating makes for the most delicious broccoli side. You won't be able to resist it, either!

1 Preheat the oven to 425°F (220°C). Line a baking sheet with parchment paper.

2 Place the broccoli florets in a large bowl. Add the oil, garlic powder, and pepper, and toss to coat. Transfer the broccoli to the baking sheet.

3 Bake for 16 to 18 minutes, until fork-tender (see Tip 2).

4 Immediately transfer the florets back to the bowl. Add the Parmesan, and toss to coat until the cheese melts.

Storage

Store in an airtight container in the fridge for up to 4 days. To reheat, microwave for 20 to 30 seconds, until warmed through.

Tips

1. Dairy-free? Swap the Parmesan with nutritional yeast.
2. If preparing this for a baby, ensure that the florets are soft and tender.

Fruity Chia Jams

prep **5 minutes** / cook **10 minutes** / makes **1½ cups (500 g)**

DF **EF** **GF** **NF** **V**

Blueberry Chia Jam

2 cups (300 g) fresh or frozen blueberries

1 tablespoon fresh lemon juice

2 tablespoons chia seeds

1 to 2 tablespoons maple syrup (optional)

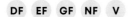

DF **EF** **GF** **NF** **V**

Raspberry Apple Jam

2 cups (300 g) fresh or frozen raspberries

½ cup (125 g) unsweetened applesauce

2 tablespoons chia seeds

1 to 2 tablespoons maple syrup (optional)

There are a few baby-friendly jarred jams on the market, but it's so easy to make your own with a few simple ingredients! These jams are sweetened with berries and thickened with chia seeds and are a great homemade alternative to store-bought jams. They're perfect for spreading on toast, stirring into yogurt, or flavoring oatmeal.

1 Heat the blueberries and lemon juice (for Blueberry Chia Jam) or raspberries and applesauce (for Raspberry Apple Jam) in a medium saucepan over medium-low heat. Allow the berries to soften and release their juices, about 5 minutes.

2 Use a fork or potato masher to mash the berries, and let them cook for an additional 5 minutes.

3 Turn off the heat, and stir in the chia seeds and maple syrup (if using). Cover the pan, and let sit for 10 minutes so the chia seeds can thicken the jam.

4 Let cool completely before serving (see Tip).

Storage

Store in an airtight container in the fridge for up to 1 week. To freeze, store in a freezer-safe container for up to 3 months.

Tip

· If you prefer a smoother jam, pass the mixture through a sieve before serving. You can also use finely ground chia seeds.

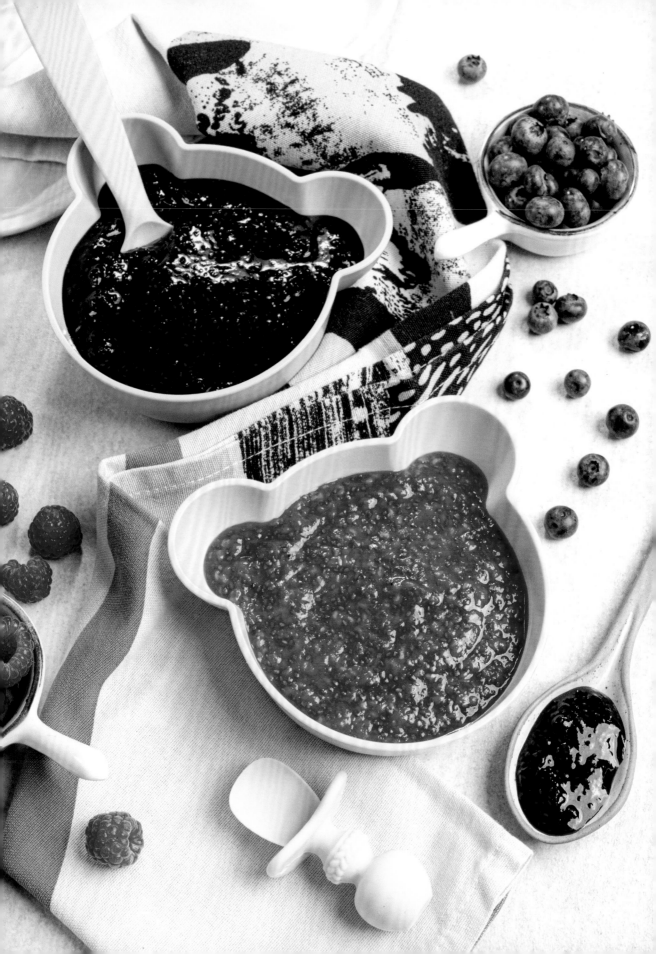

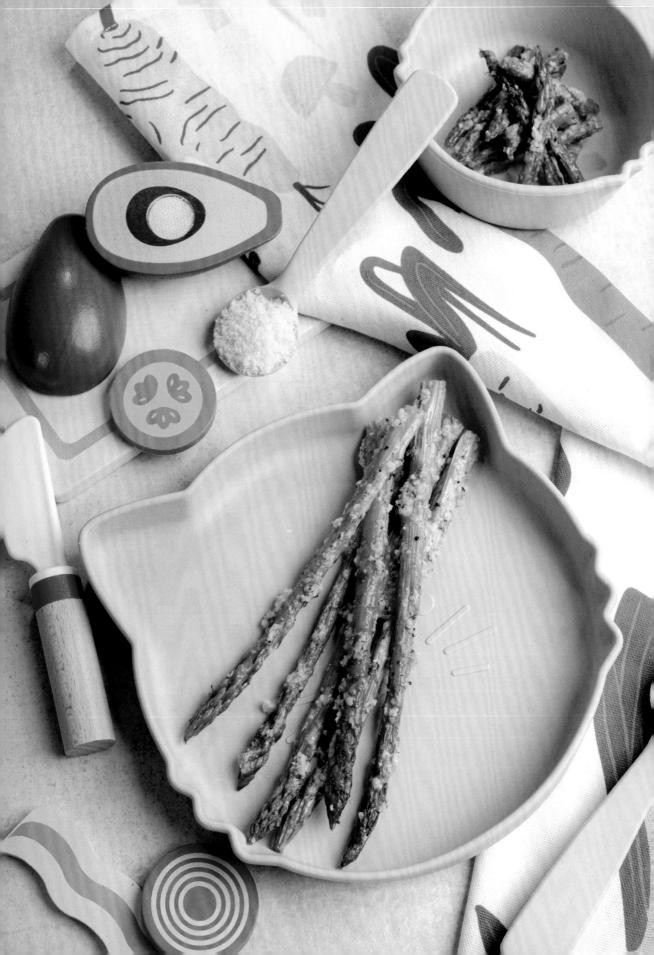

Oven-Roasted Asparagus

prep **5 minutes** / cook **15 minutes** / serves **2 adults & 1 child**

10 ounces (283 g) asparagus spears (see Tip 1)

2 tablespoons mild-tasting oil

2 tablespoons grated Parmesan (see Tip 2)

¼ teaspoon garlic powder

¼ teaspoon black pepper

Salt, to taste (optional)

I'll admit that I never was a fan of asparagus growing up. Something about the woody bottom and the stringy top seemed so unappealing to me, and I avoided it at all costs. But when my mom started roasting it in the oven with a little Parmesan, I was shocked at how tender and delicious it was! I've been making it this way ever since and have officially converted to team asparagus.

1 Preheat the oven to 425°F (220°C). Line a baking sheet with parchment paper.

2 Place the asparagus in a large bowl and drizzle the oil on top. Sprinkle on the Parmesan, garlic powder, pepper, and salt (if using) and toss to coat.

3 Place the asparagus in an even layer on the baking sheet, making sure the spears don't overlap.

4 Bake for 13 to 15 minutes, until tender.

Storage

Store in an airtight container in the fridge for up to 2 days. To reheat, microwave for 10 to 15 seconds, until warmed through.

Tips

1. If preparing this for a baby, cut off the tough bottom of the asparagus spear, and serve the top only.

2. Dairy-free? Swap the Parmesan with 1 tablespoon of nutritional yeast.

Oven-Baked Potato Wedges

prep **10 minutes** / cook **40 minutes** / serves **3 adults & 3 children**

2 pounds (907 g) red potatoes (see Tip 1)

3 tablespoons olive oil

1 teaspoon sweet paprika

½ teaspoon garlic powder

½ teaspoon onion powder

1 teaspoon salt (optional, see Tip 2)

These oven-baked potato wedges are a simple and satisfying side dish that pairs perfectly with just about any meal. Crispy on the outside and tender on the inside, these wedges are seasoned to perfection with simple spices that the whole family will love.

1 Preheat the oven to 425°F (220°C). Line a large baking sheet with parchment paper.

2 Thoroughly wash the potatoes and slice them into wedges that are ¾ inch (2 cm) thick and 4 inches (10 cm) long. Lay out the wedges, and pat them dry with paper towels to remove the excess starch.

3 Place the wedges in a large bowl. Add the oil and then sprinkle in the paprika, garlic powder, onion powder, and salt (if using). Toss to coat.

4 Transfer the wedges to the baking sheet in a single layer so they are not overlapping.

5 Bake for 35 to 40 minutes, turning them halfway through, until fork-tender and crisp on the outside.

Storage

Store in an airtight container in the fridge for up to 3 days. To reheat, place on a parchment paper–lined baking sheet, and bake in a 350°F (180°C) oven for 8 to 10 minutes, until warmed through.

Tips

1. Feel free to use russet or Yukon Gold potatoes instead.

2. If preparing this for a baby, remove baby's portion, then sprinkle the salt on the remaining potato mixture for the rest of the family. Cook baby's portion on the same baking sheet in a separate corner of the pan.

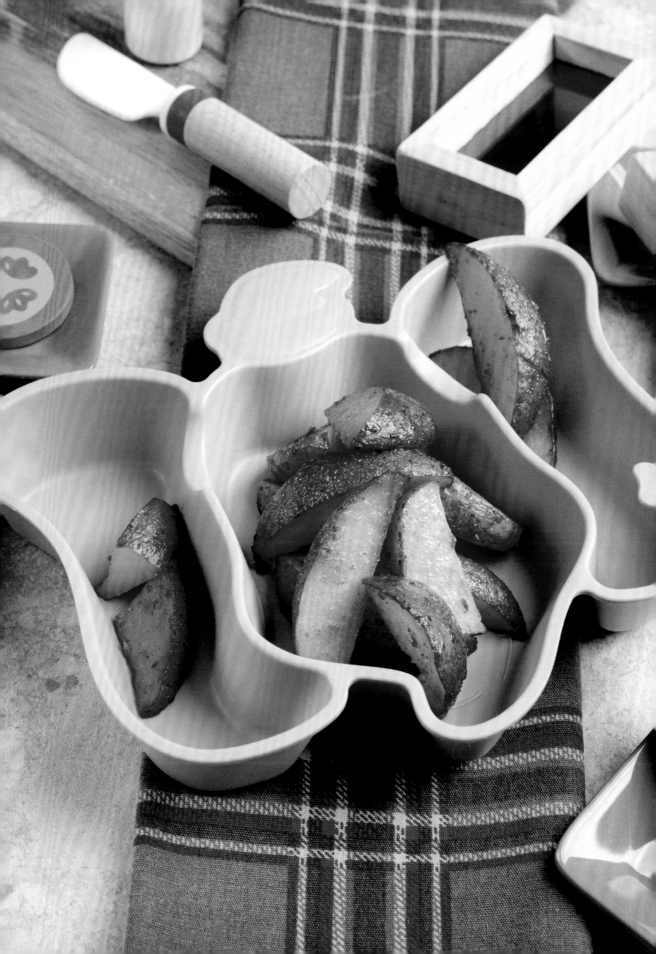

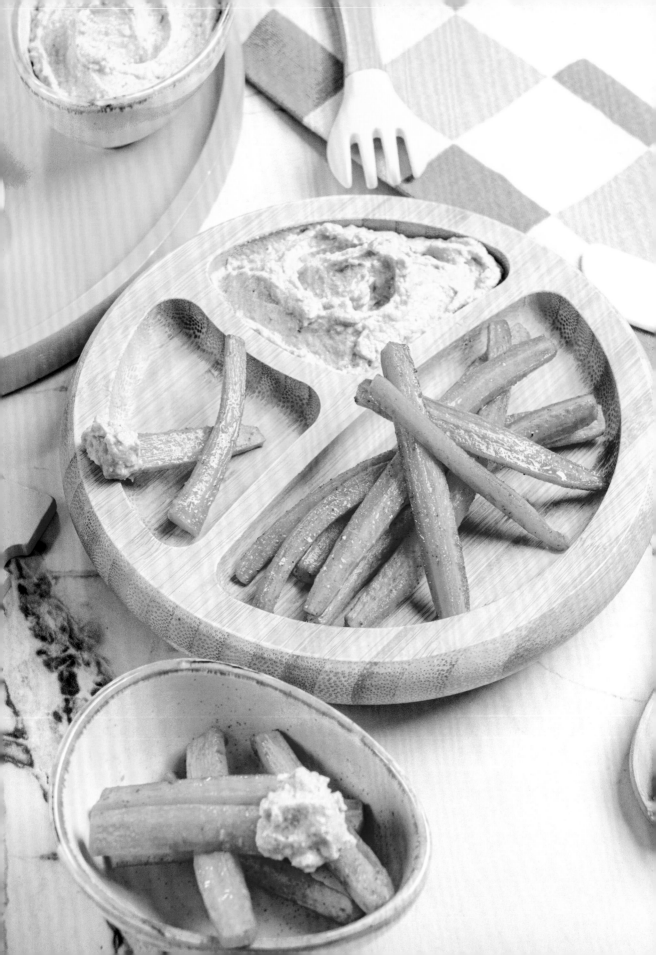

Carrot Fries & Creamy Avocado Dip

Carrot Fries

4 large carrots
1 tablespoon olive oil
½ teaspoon sweet
  paprika
¼ teaspoon salt (optional,
  see Tip 1)

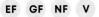

Creamy Avocado Dip

1 ripe avocado, pitted
¼ cup (55 g) cream
  cheese, softened
1 teaspoon fresh lemon
  juice (optional)
¼ teaspoon garlic
  powder
⅛ teaspoon black pepper
Salt, to taste (optional)

These carrot fries, seasoned to perfection and baked in the oven, are a fun side dish. The avocado and cream cheese in the dip pair perfectly with the fries for a flavorful, high-calorie boost for your little one! The dip is also great for spreading on toast, bagels, and crackers or as the base of any sandwich.

Carrot Fries

prep **3 minutes** / cook **25 minutes** / serves **1 adult & 2 children**

1 Preheat the oven to 400°F (200°C). Line a baking sheet with parchment paper.

2 Peel the carrots, and slice them into fry shapes.

3 Place the carrot fries in a medium bowl, and drizzle the oil over the top. Add the paprika and salt (if using), and toss to coat. Place the carrots in an even layer in the baking pan.

4 Bake for 22 to 25 minutes, shaking halfway through, until fork-tender (see Tip 2).

Creamy Avocado Dip

prep **3 minutes** / makes **1 cup (230 g)**

1 Scoop the avocado flesh into a medium bowl. Mash with a fork until smooth.

2 Add the cream cheese, lemon juice, garlic powder, black pepper, and salt (if using), and mix until smooth.

Storage

Store leftover carrot fries in an airtight container in the fridge for up to 3 days. To reheat, place the fries on a parchment paper–lined baking sheet, and bake in a 350°F (180°C) oven for 8 to 10 minutes, until warmed through. The avocado dip is best served fresh but can be stored in an airtight container in the fridge for up to 2 days.

Tips

1. If preparing these for a baby, remove baby's portion and sprinkle salt on the rest, making sure to toss to coat.
2. Prefer to air-fry? Place the fries in an even layer on an air-fryer basket, and air-fry at 400°F (200°C) for 12 to 15 minutes, shaking the basket halfway through.

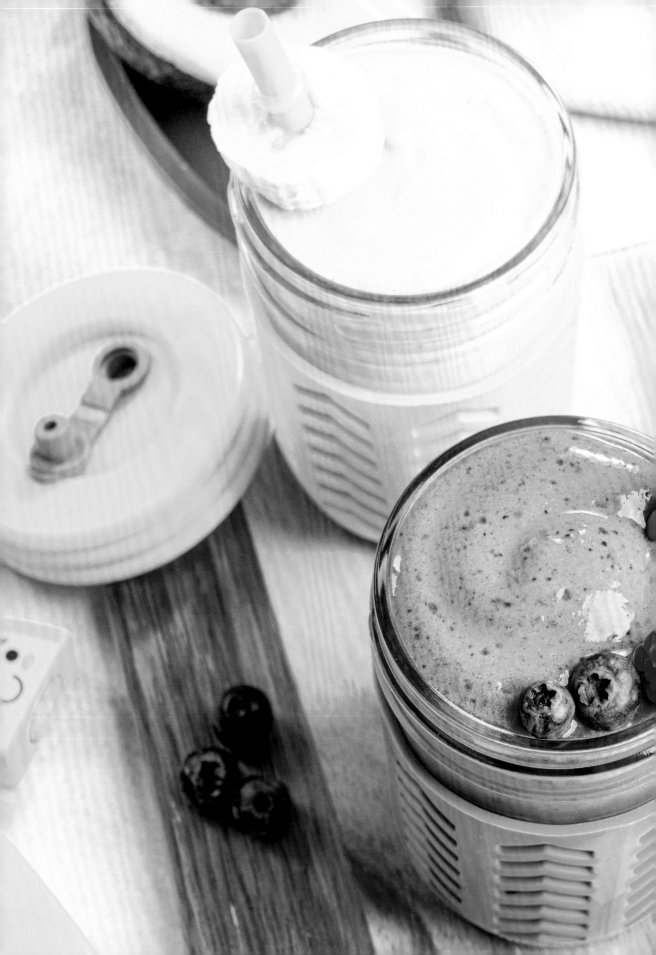

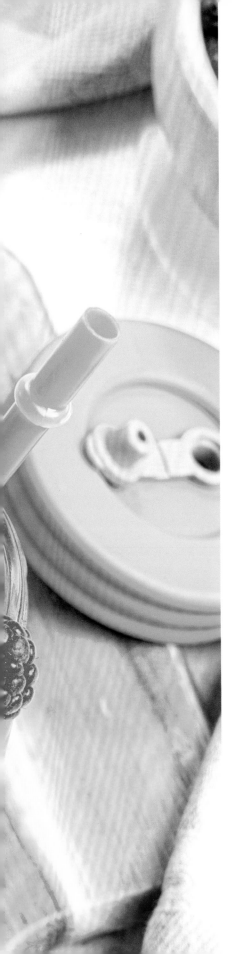

Refreshing Drinks

Smoothies and shakes are always a great option to serve little ones to keep them refreshed and hydrated. This chapter contains some of my favorite drink recipes made with fruits, veggies, and healthy fats as another way to get in some of those nutrients throughout the day. Keep in mind that if your little one is under the age of one, breast milk and formula should be the primary beverage and source of nutrition.

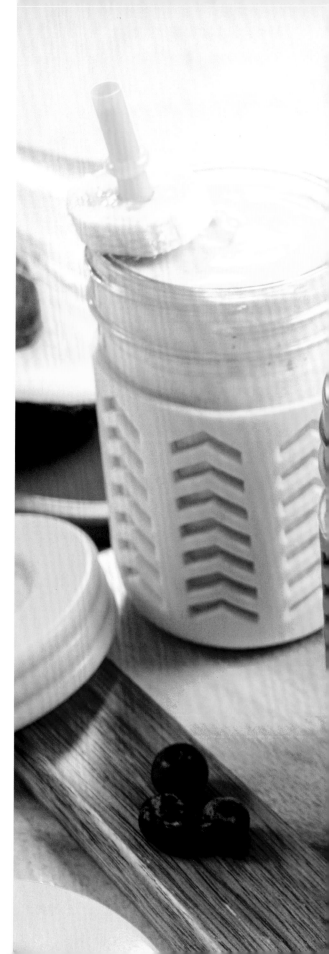

Avocado Banana Smoothie

prep **5 minutes** / serves **1 adult & 1 child**

This smoothie is thick and creamy, perfect first thing in the morning or as a snack. It's packed with healthy fats and is a fun, bright color your little one is sure to love!

2 small (or 1½ large) overripe bananas
1 medium ripe avocado
2 tablespoons natural peanut butter (see Tip 1)
1 cup (240 ml) milk
5 to 6 ice cubes

1 Add the ingredients to a blender, and blend until smooth (see Tips 2 and 3).

2 Pour into cups to serve.

Storage

This milkshake is best enjoyed fresh but can be frozen for up to 1 month and thawed for later use.

Tips

1. Nut-free? Swap the peanut butter with a seed-based butter, or omit it completely.

2. Blend in some ground flaxseed for an added nutritional boost!

3. If your smoothie is a little thick, blend in a few more splashes of milk to thin it out.

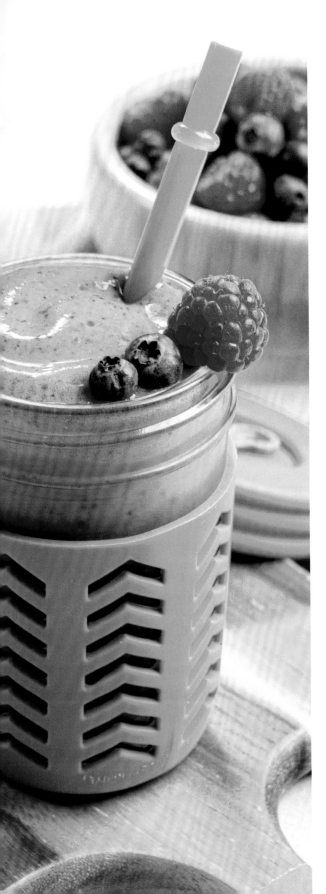

Beet Berry Smoothie

prep **5 minutes** / serves **1 adult & 1 child**

Beets are loaded with vitamins and minerals but often get a bad rap because many people aren't fans of the earthy taste. When combined with mixed berries, though, they create this delicious, creamy drink. Not to mention their beautiful, vivid color!

1 cup (150 g) frozen mixed berries (see Tip)
½ cup (80 g) precooked beets
¾ cup (160 g) plain whole milk Greek yogurt
¼ cup (60 ml) milk
1 tablespoon ground flaxseeds
1 tablespoon maple syrup (optional)

1 Add the frozen mixed berries, beets, yogurt, milk, flaxseeds, and maple syrup (if using) to a blender, and blend until smooth.

2 Pour into cups to serve.

Storage

This smoothie is best enjoyed fresh but can be frozen for up to 1 month and thawed for later use.

Tip

- If you don't have frozen mixed berries on hand, replace them with frozen blueberries, strawberries, or any other berries!

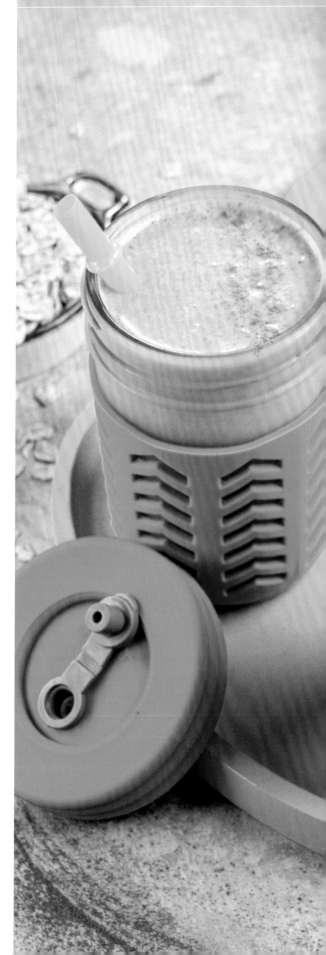

EF GF V

Spinach Banana Smoothie

prep **5 minutes** / serves **1 adult & 1 child**

This "Hulk smoothie" is not only a fun green color but also a balanced breakfast or snack! It's made with rolled oats, which will help keep your little one full. When my little guys aren't in the mood for a full breakfast, or when I'm looking for a filling snack to help get them through to dinnertime, a smoothie is always a go-to. Rolled oats are packed with fiber and whole grains, and peanut butter contains protein and healthy fats for a well-balanced treat.

2 small (or 1½ large) overripe bananas
¼ cup (23 g) old-fashioned rolled oats
¾ cups (180 ml) milk
2 tablespoons natural peanut butter (see Tip)
¼ cup (15 g) spinach, packed
¼ teaspoon ground cinnamon
5 to 6 ice cubes

1 Add the ingredients to a blender, and blend until smooth.

2 Pour into cups to serve.

Storage

This smoothie is best enjoyed fresh but can be frozen for up to 1 month and thawed for later use.

Tip

· Nut-free? Swap the peanut butter with a seed-based butter, or omit it completely.

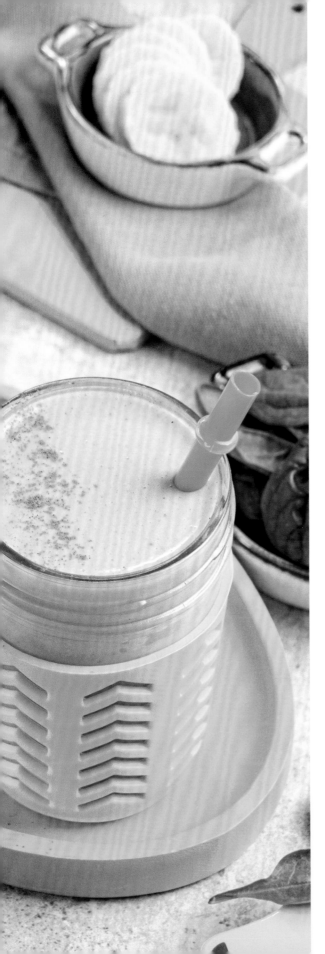

Sweet Potato Smoothie

prep **5 minutes** / serves **1 adult & 1 child**

This smoothie tastes like your favorite slice of sweet potato pie in drink form. It is naturally sweetened with sweet potatoes and banana and has a touch of warm spice flavor from the cinnamon. Whenever I have leftover sweet potatoes, I save them to turn into this smoothie.

½ cup (120 g) mashed cooked sweet potato (see Tip 1)
1 large ripe banana
½ cup (120 ml) milk
½ cup (120 g) plain whole milk Greek yogurt
1 tablespoon natural peanut butter (see Tip 2)
½ teaspoon ground cinnamon
5 to 6 ice cubes

1 Add the ingredients to a blender, and blend until smooth.

2 Pour into cups to serve.

Storage

This smoothie is best enjoyed fresh but can be frozen for up to 1 month and thawed for later use.

Tips

1. You may precook sweet potatoes in the oven (poke holes in the potatoes, and bake at 425°F/220°C for 45 to 50 minutes, until tender) or in the microwave (poke holes in the potatoes, and microwave for 5 to 6 minutes, until tender). Let cool, then peel and mash.

2. Nut-free? Swap the peanut butter with a seed-based butter, or omit it completely.

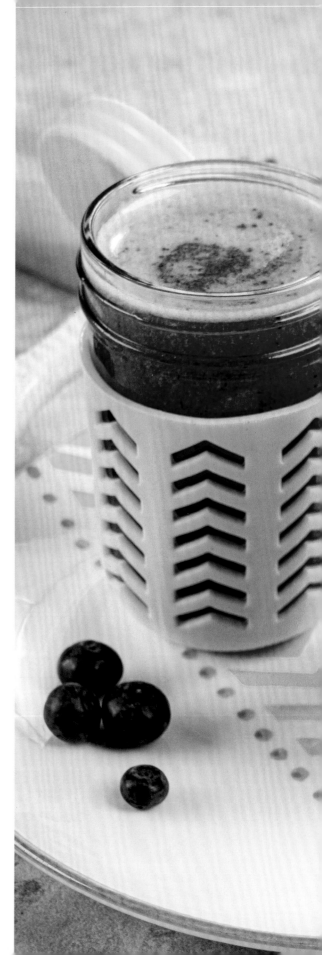

Blueberry Lemonade

prep **5 minutes** / serves **1 adult & 1 child**

There's nothing like a fresh cup of ice-cold lemonade on a hot day. My boys have never hosted an official lemonade stand, but if they ever do, they'll definitely serve this fruity drink!

1 cup (150 g) fresh blueberries
¼ cup (60 ml) fresh lemon juice
2 tablespoons maple syrup

1 In a blender, blend together the blueberries and 1 cup (240 ml) of water. Strain through a sieve into a pitcher (see Tip 1).

2 Add another 1 cup (240 ml) of water, the lemon juice, and maple syrup to the blueberry mixture, and stir until well combined (see Tip 2).

3 Serve chilled over ice.

Storage

This lemonade is best enjoyed fresh but can be stored in the fridge for 1 day. Be sure to give it a good stir before serving because some of the mixture may settle to the bottom.

Tips

1. If you don't mind blueberry chunks in the drink, you can skip the straining step.
2. Feel free to adjust the lemonade to taste. Add a little more maple syrup for additional sweetness, more lemon juice for extra tartness, or more water to balance out the flavors as needed.

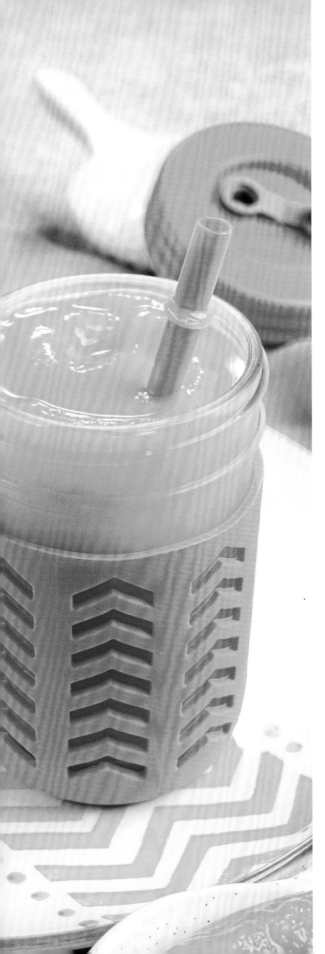

Peach Slush

prep **5 minutes** / serves **1 adult & 1 child**

Homemade slushies are a summertime favorite in our home. They're so refreshing and a great way to stay hydrated on hot days. I use canned peaches as a quick option, but you can use fresh or frozen peaches as you like.

One 15-ounce (425 g) can unsweetened sliced peaches, drained (or 1¼ cups/255 g sliced peaches)
1 cup (150 g) frozen mango chunks
Juice of ½ lime
5 to 6 ice cubes

1 Add the ingredients to a blender, and blend until smooth (see Tip).

2 Pour into cups to serve.

Storage

This smoothie is best enjoyed fresh but can be frozen for up to 1 month and thawed for later use.

Tip

· If you prefer a sweeter drink, blend in 1 tablespoon of maple syrup.

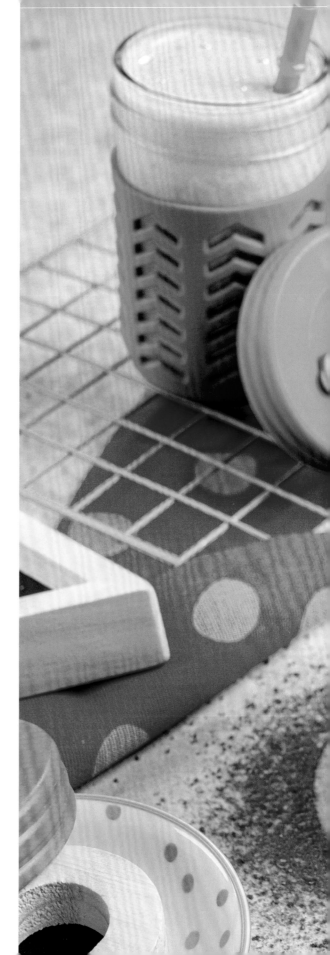

EF GF NF V

Strawberry Milkshake

prep **5 minutes** / serves **1 adult & 1 child**

This strawberry milkshake comes together with only a few ingredients for a refreshing, sweet drink. The cauliflower—yes, cauliflower!—provides extra creaminess and added veggie nutrition, but the strawberry flavor is what comes through.

1 cup (150 g) diced strawberries
1 cup (240 ml) milk
¼ cup (35 g) frozen riced cauliflower (see Tip 1)
2 teaspoons maple syrup (optional)

1 Add the strawberries, milk, cauliflower, and maple syrup (if using) to a blender, and blend until smooth (see Tip 2).

2 Pour into cups to serve.

Storage

This milkshake is best enjoyed fresh but can be frozen for up to 1 month and thawed for later use.

Tips

1. If you only have fresh riced cauliflower, you can add a couple of ice cubes to keep the shake cold.
2. Blend in some hemp hearts for an added nutritional boost!

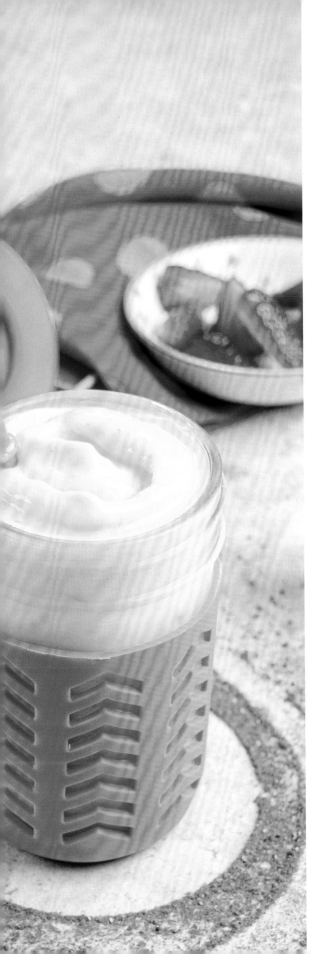

Mango Apple Drinkable Yogurt

prep **5 minutes** / serves **1 adult & 1 child**

Yogurt drinks are a fun way to serve up some protein and calcium, but those little bottles at the store can get so expensive! This method uses yogurt, milk, and fruit to make DIY yogurt drinks in just 5 minutes! You can swap out the fruits as you like for different flavor combinations.

1 cup (150 g) frozen mango chunks
1 cup (250 g) unsweetened applesauce
½ cup (120 g) plain whole milk Greek yogurt
½ cup (120 ml) milk
1 tablespoon maple syrup (optional)

1 Add the mango, applesauce, yogurt, milk, and maple syrup (if using) to a blender, and blend until smooth (see Tips 1 and 2).

2 Pour into cups to serve.

Storage

This drinkable yogurt is best enjoyed fresh but can be frozen for up to 1 month and thawed for later use.

Tips

1. Blend in some hemp hearts for an added nutritional boost!
2. If your yogurt drink is a little thick, blend in a few more splashes of milk to thin it out.

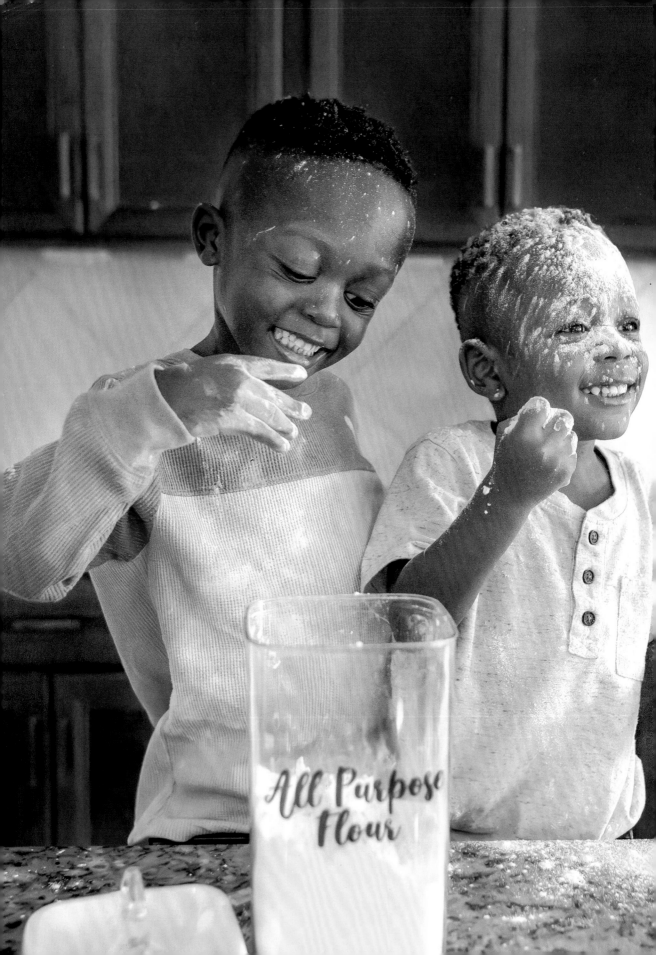

Notes

1 US Department of Agriculture and US Department of Health and Human Services, *Dietary Guidelines for Americans, 2020–2025*, 9th ed., December 2020. https://www.dietaryguidelines.gov/sites/default/files/2020-12/Dietary_Guidelines_for_Americans_2020-2025.pdf.

2 "Foods and Drinks to Avoid or Limit," Centers for Disease Control and Prevention, April 19, 2024, https://www.cdc.gov/nutrition/infantandtoddlernutrition/foods-and-drinks/foods-and-drinks-to-limit.html.

3 Amy Brown, "No Difference in Self-Reported Frequency of Choking Between Infants Introduced to Solid Foods Using a Baby-Led Weaning or Traditional Spoon-Feeding Approach," *Journal of Human Nutrition and Dietetics* 31, no. 4 (2017): 496–504, https://doi.org/10.1111/jhn.12528.

4 "Choking Hazards," Centers for Disease Control and Prevention, February 25, 2022, https://www.cdc.gov/nutrition/infantandtoddlernutrition/foods-and-drinks/choking-hazards.html.

5 Steve Schering, "Follow Safety Advice When Preparing Meats for Young Children," *AAP News*, June 1, 2022, https://publications.aap.org/aapnews/news/20241/Follow-safety-advice-when-preparing-meats-for.

6 Mohamed H. Abd El-Salam and Safinaz El-Shibiny, "Reduction of Milk Protein Antigenicity by Enzymatic Hydrolysis and Fermentation. A Review," *Food Reviews International* 37, no. 3 (2019): 276–95, https://doi.org/10.1080/87559129.2019.1701010.

7 Waheeda Samady et al., "Recommendations on Complementary Food Introduction Among Pediatric Practitioners," *JAMA Network Open* 3, no. 8, e2013070, (2020): https://doi.org/10.1001/jamanetworkopen.2020.13070.

8 Edmond S. Chan and Carl Cummings, "Dietary Exposures and Allergy Prevention in High-Risk Infants," *Paediatrics & Child Health* 18, no. 10 (2013): 545–49, https://doi.org/10.1093/pch/18.10.545.

9 Elissa M. Abrams, et al., "Updates in Food Allergy Prevention in Children," *Pediatrics* 152, no. 5 (2023): e2023062836, https://doi.org/10.1542/peds.2023-062836.

10 "Salt in Your Diet," National Health Service, April 17, 2023, https://www.nhs.uk/live-well/eat-well/food-types/salt-in-your-diet.

11 Jill Rabin, MS, CCC-SLP/L IBCLC, Instagram message to author, May 25, 2023.

12 Catherine A. Forestell and Julie A. Mennella, "Early Determinants of Fruit and Vegetable Acceptance," *Pediatrics* 120, no. 6 (2007): 1247–54, https://doi.org/10.1542/peds.2007-0858.

Index

oats

pan-fried

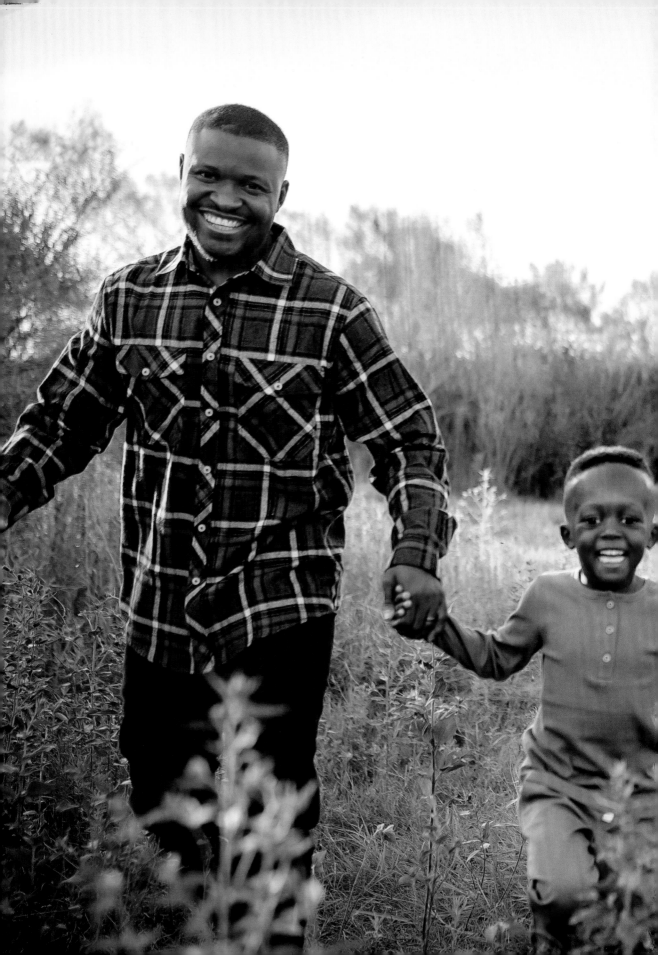

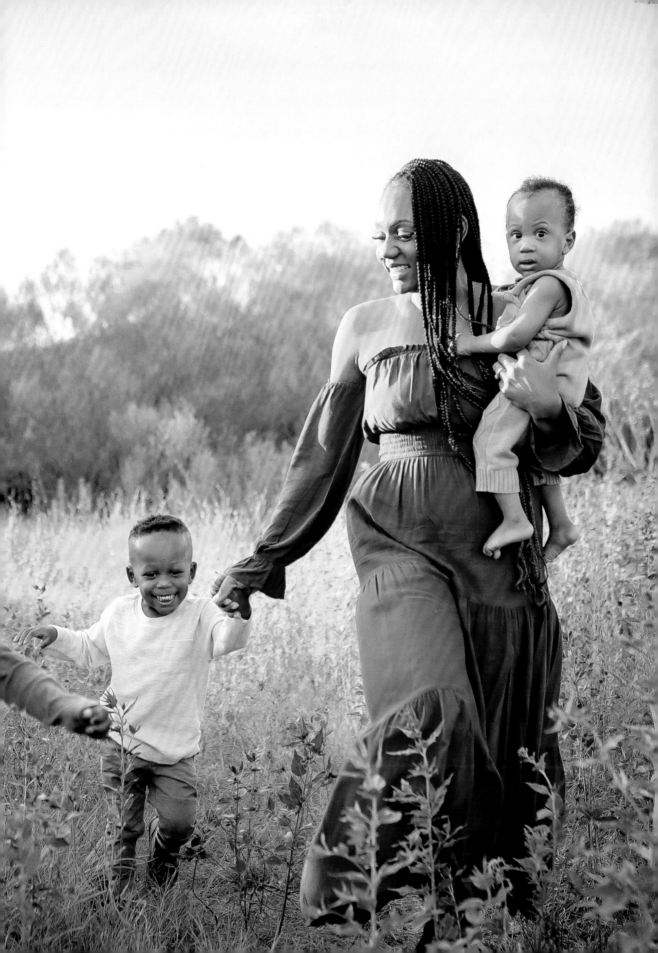

Acknowledgments

To the supporters of the Feeding Tiny Bellies online community: This book is for you! Thank you for your unwavering support of our family and for trying our recipes. You've inspired me to write this book, and I hope that it brings you much inspiration. It gives me so much joy to see your families enjoying the recipes, and I hope this book serves as a valuable tool for you. You are the reason I do what I do, and I am so grateful for you all.

To my husband, Florince: Thank you for supporting me on this journey. This book would never have happened had you not encouraged me to start a blog and supported me every step of the way. Your love pushed me to work diligently and put my all into this project. Thank you for willingly taste testing every single recipe in this book. Even when you were stuffed and couldn't take another bite, you always made room for another sample because you knew that I wanted your feedback. Thank you for always keeping me company while I made the kitchen a mess every day and for having mini dance parties with me as we cleaned up together at night. This book is exactly what I envisioned because of you, my biggest cheerleader.

To my sons, Myles, Levi, and Kai: Thank you for being the best sons I could ever ask for. Your honest feedback on recipes always makes me laugh, from your "This isn't good, Mama" comments to your "This one is yummy!" praise. I'm so grateful to have you all be part of the taste-testing team. I will always cherish the time we've spent together in the kitchen, and I feel blessed to have you all as my little sous-chefs.

To my dear parents: Thank you for willingly flying out countless times to come visit and care for the boys so I could have time to test recipes and write for this project. The boys are so fortunate to have such amazing grandparents who genuinely love them, and I'm grateful to be able to call you Mom and Dad.

To my incredible editor, Olivia: Thank you for being so communicative and detail-oriented throughout this project. You went above and beyond to ensure that every single word of this book was edited to perfection, and I truly appreciate your guidance, input, and support.

To the entire team at DK Publishing: Thank you for choosing me to write this book and believing that I had a story to tell. I couldn't have asked for a more supportive team to bring this book to fruition.

To my agent, Sally Ekus: Thank you for taking me under your wing to bring this project to life. You were always there when I had questions along the way and believed in my vision from the start.

To my dear friend Min Jun: Thank you for agreeing to work with me on this book. I am so thankful to have you as the registered dietitian to review the informational content in this book, ensuring that all the content and advice are nutritionally sound and align with up-to-date research. Your input has been invaluable!

And most importantly, to my Heavenly Father: Thank you for giving me the strength and energy to persevere when writing this book. I prayed to you countless times when I encountered roadblocks, and I am in constant awe of your mercy and grace.

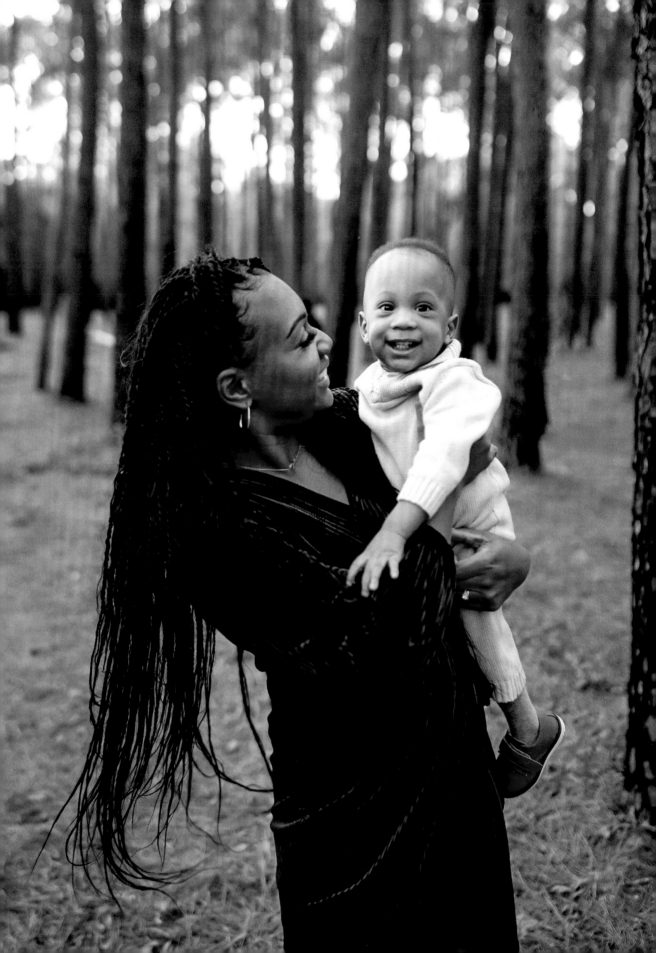

About the Author

Lily Payen is a recipe developer and founder of Feeding Tiny Bellies, a website she created as a way to share simple and nutritious recipes for busy parents to make for their little ones. She has bachelor's and master's degrees in mathematics and is a former secondary education teacher. There is so much math involved in cooking, and her math expertise helps her determine precise measurements and ratios that work to create simple, nutritious recipes. She lives with her husband and three children in Houston, Texas.

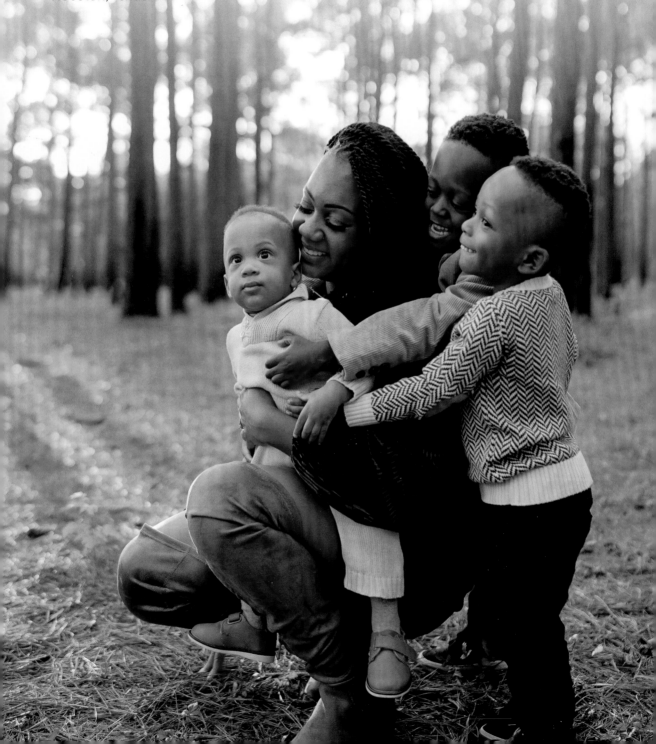